P9-DCJ-489

KF
3826
.E5
M36

EMERGENCY CARE AND THE LAW

Marguerite R. Mancini
and
Alice T. Gale

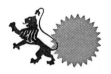

AN ASPEN PUBLICATION®
Aspen Systems Corporation
Rockville, Maryland
London
1981

Tennessee Tech. Library
Cookeville, Tenn.
310201

Library of Congress Cataloging in Publication Data

Mancini, Marguerite R.
Emergency care and the law.

Includes index.
1. Emergency medical services— Law and legislation—
United States. I. Gale, Alice T. II. Title.
[DNLM: 1. Emergency service, Hospital— Legislation.
WX 33.1 M269e]
KF3826.E5M36   346.7303'1   81-4364
ISBN: 0-89443-337-7   347.30631   AACR2

Copyright © 1981 Aspen Systems Corporation

All rights reserved. This book, or parts thereof, may not be
reproduced in any form or by any means, electronic or
mechanical, including photocopy, recording, or any
information storage and retrieval system now known or
to be invented, without written permission from the
publisher, except in the case of brief quotations embodied
in critical articles or reviews. For information, address
Aspen Systems Corporation, 1600 Research Boulevard,
Rockville, Maryland 20850.

Library of Congress Catalog Card Number: 81-4364
ISBN: 0-89443-337-7

Printed in the United States of America

1 2 3 4 5

To my daughters, *Janet and Karen,* who have always been a source of encouragement to me and who gave their assistance to the completion of this book.

— MRM

To *George, Nancy, and George*

— ATG

Table of Contents

Preface

In the past few decades, the use of emergency rooms in general hospitals by the public has increased dramatically. This increase shows no sign of abating at the present time. Many legal questions confront those health care professionals—nurses, doctors, and hospital administrators—whose practices involve them in providing emergency health care. The nature of emergency care seldom allows for lengthy deliberation in making treatment decisions. A good number of these decisions have legal ramifications.

This book is written primarily as an aid to health care professionals and students who practice in emergency health care settings. It is designed to explain legal principles and their application to the provision of emergency health care. Specific issues of concern in the delivery of emergency health care are highlighted, and case illustrations demonstrate how the courts look at facts to reach decisions. By being informed of how the law interfaces with emergency health care, involved practitioners may not only prevent problems of liability, but allow themselves to concentrate on doing what they do best: providing good health care on an acute basis.

This book can be used as a general legal guide to emergency health care. It should not be used carelessly for specific answers to specific situations. Local counsel should always be consulted for advice about a particular set of facts.

Part I

Introduction to Emergency Room Law

Chapter 1

An Overview of the Law

The law, as it applies to the functioning of emergency rooms in U.S. hospitals, is a relatively new area of specialization for attorneys. In 1973 the American Bar Association first recognized the specialty of Health Care and Hospital Law.

This is not to say that this specialty is practiced any differently from any other area of the law; it is not. However, because the focus of any hospital emergency room is the health and well-being of citizens, there are specific aspects that often are not seen in other legal specialties. To understand how legal principles are applied to health care in general and to emergency health care in particular, it is important to first review some basic legal concepts.

American law is taken from the English system of law brought to this country by the colonists. In the United States we use both common law and statutory law. Both have application to health care in general and to emergency care in particular.

COMMON LAW

Common law, also called case law, is judge-made rather than legislature-enacted. It is the law of judicial decisions. An example of common law is the law of informed consent. Recently there has been some movement by states such as Massachusetts to enact statutes that address the issue of consent to treatment. This is a new trend, however, and is a general exception to the common law doctrine of informed consent.

One important principle of common law is the notion of precedent. A judicial decision serves two purposes: it settles or resolves a dispute, and it establishes a precedent to guide the resolution of similar situations that are brought to court at some future date. *Stare decisis* is the common law principle of following precedent in resolving disputes in court. Precedent allows for legal stability by prohibiting courts from changing legal rules at whim. It also allows for predictability in that it permits interested parties to study how courts have handled similar situations in the past.

Common law should not be seen as totally stationary, however. The common law has the capacity to grow and reflect advances in knowledge and thinking; law is rewritten when earlier judicial decisions are clearly outdated.

STATUTORY LAW

Statutory law refers to acts of law dictated by the legislative branch of government. Typically, statutory law declares, commands, or prohibits something. A statute is the written will of the legislature, solemnly expressed according to those forms necessary to constitute it as the law of the state. One example of statutory law would be state laws that govern and regulate the practice of professions such as nursing and medicine.

Statutory law is thus enacted and written in codes of state and federal laws. As it applies to and defines the practice of the professions, statutory law broadly and generally states what the professional is legally allowed to do.

REGULATIONS AND POLICIES

Regulations, although neither judge-made nor legislature-enacted, have the force of law because they are the rulings of a governmental agency. Regulations are issued by a department head under an act of Congress or on the authority of a state legislature that confers the necessary power and thereby gives such regulations legal force. The authority given to the agency head to issue regulations is delegated power; the power is delegated by the legislative body.

Regulations specifically define areas of legislation and are written to implement statutes. Regulations written to implement a law cannot go beyond the law by addressing areas not included in the original legislation.

Policies, as opposed to laws, are the internal rules and regulations of an institution. To illustrate, in most health care institutions, policies are formulated by medical boards and by administration. The policy-making body is usually the board of directors or board of trustees. It is the duty and responsibility of the administrators to implement policy. The power of implementation is delegated to the administrators by the governing body.

In legal terms, laws, regulations, and policies do exist simultaneously. Problems arise when they are in conflict. The law is clear on which governs in the face of conflict. If a statute conflicts with a regulation, the statute governs. If a policy conflicts with a regulation, the regulation governs.

The governing board of a health institution or facility has general authority to manage the business. This authority is absolute so long as the board acts within the law. The courts leave questions of policy and internal management to the discretion of the governing boards.

Inherent in the management function is the authority of the governing board to set policies for the institution. The board may exercise this policy-making authority or delegate it to the administration. The delegation may be broad or narrow. In some cases the governing board may choose to set or delegate a broad range of power, covering general policies plus policies specific to a particular department. Or the board may choose to set the overall policies but delegate responsibility for setting policies that pertain to particular subdivisions or departments, such as the emergency room.

Hospitals, with or without emergency departments, must function within the law. Thus hospitals must follow all state laws and regulations that apply directly to hospitals. If they are recipients of federal funding, they are also subject to all applicable federal laws and regulations. All states now require hospitals to be licensed, whether they are private or public corporations, nonprofit or proprietary.

CRIMINAL AND TORT LAW

A crime is a positive or negative act in violation of the penal law, an offense against the state. Crime may be defined as any act done in violation of those duties that an individual owes to the community, for the breach of which the law has provided that the offender shall make satisfaction to the public. A crime is distinguished from a tort or civil injury in that the former is considered a breach and violation of public rights and responsibilities as seen in the context of the whole community, whereas the latter is an infringement or privation of the rights of individuals as opposed to the state. A criminal act can be prosecuted only by the state; an individual cannot prosecute for a criminal act. In tort law, suit is brought by one or more individuals against one or more individuals. Normally the state is not involved.

In criminal law, the offender is punished with fines or imprisonment— sometimes (but with less and less frequency) even death. In criminal law the punishment is aligned with deterrence. In civil or tort law, the punishment is aligned with compensating the victim for his or her loss. Because fines and imprisonment would not accomplish this purpose, the usual punishment in civil law is compensation to the victim in the form of money damages.

Examples of criminal law offenses are acts of murder, rape, and larceny. The best example of a civil law offense in health care is malpractice, an unintentional tort. Torts can also be intentional, but in general these are rare—and certainly rare in health care.

Although most incidents that raise the issue of professional liability concern harm that allegedly results from negligence, health professionals may also be liable for intentional wrongs. In the context of patient care, intentional tortious conduct (that is, conduct implying a civil wrong) may include assault, battery, false imprisonment, invasion of privacy, libel, and slander. In health care, suits for assault and battery and for false imprisonment are more common than the others.

There are two major differences between intentional and negligent wrongs. One involves the element of intent to wrong, which is present in intentional wrongs but not in negligent wrongs. The second difference is less obvious. An intentional wrong always involves a willful act that violates another's rights; a negligent wrong may not involve any act at all. In a situation involving negligence, a person may be held liable for not acting in the way a reasonable and prudent person would have acted. Thus, negligence can involve a failure to act as well as a careless act; it can involve an act of omission or an act of commission.

An assault is an intentional act designed to place another person in apprehension of a battery. A battery is an intentional, unconsented touching of another's person. Liability for these wrongs is based on an individual's right to be free from invasion of his or her person. When an assault and/or a battery occurs, the injured person's rights have been invaded. The law provides that person with a remedy for the interference: the injured person can sue the wrongdoer for the damages suffered. Even in situations where benefits are incurred or no actual harm results, the law presumes a compensable injury to the person by virtue of the fact that the assault and/or battery occurred.

In the context of health care, the legal principles that relate to assault and battery are of critical importance. Liability of hospitals, physicians, and nurses for acts of assault and battery is most common in situations involving patient consent to medical and surgical procedures. It is inevitable that any hospital patient will be touched by many persons for many reasons. Procedures ranging from surgery to the taking of x-rays all involve some touching of the patient. Even the administration of some medications may entail touching. Therefore, medical and surgical procedures must be authorized by the patient. If they are not authorized, the person performing those procedures will be subject to an action for battery.

It is of little legal significance that the procedure in question has actually improved the patient's health. If there was no patient consent, the patient may be entitled to damages. In *Mohr* v. *Williams*, 95 Minn. 516, 104 N.W. 12 (1905), the patient consented to surgery on her right ear. When the patient was anesthetized and the physician could examine her better, he discovered that the left ear was in a more serious condition than the right ear. The patient, however, had not consented to surgery on the left ear. The physician nevertheless operated on the left ear. A judgment of $39 was awarded to the patient after a second trial. There was no assault since the patient was asleep and could not have been placed in apprehension of an unwanted touching. There was a battery because surgery had been performed on the left ear, an unwanted touching to which there had been no consent.

Issues of assault and battery involving lack of consent to treatment will be dealt with comprehensively in Chapter 4.

False imprisonment is the unlawful restraint of an individual's personal liberty, or the unlawful detention of an individual. The actual use of physical force is not necessary to constitute a false imprisonment. A reasonable fear that force—which may be implied by words, threats, or gestures—will be used to detain the individual is sufficient.

Refusing to allow a patient to leave a hospital until all bills have been paid may constitute false imprisonment. However, hospitals are not liable for false imprisonment when they compel a patient with a contagious disease to stay in the hospital. Mentally ill patients may also be kept in the hospital if there is a danger that they will take their own lives or jeopardize the lives of others. But mental illness alone is not sufficient reason to detain a patient. Patients who are mentally ill or insane can be restrained only if they present a danger to themselves or to others.

Issues of false imprisonment involving refusal to allow patients to leave the hospital are discussed more fully in Chapter 7.

JOINT COMMISSION ON ACCREDITATION OF HOSPITALS

There is one national accrediting association which, although not a legal entity, does have accreditation standards. The Joint Commission on Accreditation of Hospitals (JCAH) is a private accrediting agency. This organization inspects hospitals and accredits those that meet the association's criteria. From a legal and fiscal standpoint, the importance of accreditation is that a JCAH-accredited hospital is automatically eligible for Medicare certification as a reimbursable provider under federal regulations. In addition, the hospital must also comply with federal requirements for utilization review.

JCAH has published standards for the emergency services in hospitals. Under its standards every JCAH-accredited hospital should have a plan for emergency care. One of the standards—Standard IV—directly addresses the issue of policies. This standard requires written policies supported by procedure manuals and reference material. There is a requirement that emergency room policies be reviewed periodically, revised when necessary, and approved by the medical staff and management. JCAH also suggests that procedures be developed from the policies.

The JCAH standards for emergency services are summarized as follows:[1]

Standard I.—"A well-defined plan for emergency care, based on community need and on the capability of the hospital, shall exist within every hospital."

Whether the hospital operates no emergency service, a limited emergency service, or a full emergency service, the hospital must have some procedure whereby the emergency patient can be assessed and given "essential life-saving measures and provide(d) emergency procedures that will minimize aggravation of the condition during transportation."

The receiving institution must consent to accept the patient before transfer can take place. A reasonable medical record of the immediate medical problem must accompany the patient. Hospitals in a community should identify the readiness of each hospital and staff to receive and treat all emergency patients.

Standard II.—"The emergency service, when maintained, shall be well organized, properly directed, and integrated with other departments of the hospital. Staffing shall be related to the scope and nature of the needs anticipated and the services offered."

There must be an organizational plan that identifies the emergency service and its relationship to other departments within the hospital and to other community emergency services. There should be someone who acts as a chief of emergency services. Service must be available 24 hours a day, and coverage by medical staff must be adequate to ensure that an emergency patient will be seen within a reasonable length of time and that any necessary laboratory work will be carried out promptly. "(S)pecialists in limited practice shall be available on an established schedule for consultation and special services in response to the needs of the emergency patient." There should be an adequate number of nurses for the amount and type of care to be provided. These nurses should have been specially trained. Physicians, nurses, and all allied health personnel "shall" be required to have cardiopulmonary resuscitative training. The hospital should provide emergency care conferences for ambulance personnel, emergency service personnel, and medical staff.

Standard III.—"Facilities for the emergency service shall be such as to ensure effective care of the patient."

The emergency service area should be near the emergency entrance and should be easily accessible from within the hospital. The receiving area should be unobstructed, and the service area should have adequate space. Enough reception, examination, treatment, and observation rooms should be provided to ensure effective patient care. Because of the many different diseases that pass through this area, procedures should be designed to eliminate the possibility of contamination and cross-infection. It is preferable that there be separate rooms for urgent limited surgery and for the treatment of fractures; there should also be a separate area for severely traumatized patients.

Instruments and supplies (such as drugs, plasma substitutes, etc.) must be on hand for immediate use. "Suction and oxygen equipment and cardiopulmonary resuscitation units must be available and ready for use" and must be suitable for adults, children, and infants. Clinical and radiological laboratory facilities should be available at all times, and patients should be escorted for tests and radiological services whenever necessary.

If possible, emergency personnel should prepare in advance for the arrival of a critical patient. This preparation can be aided by a communications system between hospital personnel and persons at the scene of the accident or in the ambulance. There also must be a separate, rapid communications system that connects the emergency service with all functionally related areas of the hospital, including the blood storage area, the surgical suite, clinical laboratories, and diagnostic radiology.

Standard IV—"Emergency patient care shall be guided by written policies and shall be supported by appropriate procedure manuals and reference material."

Policies governing the extent of treatment to be carried out in the emergency room must be periodically reviewed, revised when necessary, and approved by the medical staff and the hospital management. Procedures should be developed from the policies.

Current toxicology reference material "shall" be readily available, as well as the telephone number of the regional poison control center. Charts concerning the initial treatment of burns, cardiopulmonary resuscitation, and tetanus immunization should be on display.

Standard V.—"A medical record shall be kept for every patient receiving emergency service; it shall become an official hospital record."

The record must contain adequate patient identification, the time and means of arrival and by whom transported, the history of the injury or illness (including first aid administered prior to arrival at the hospital), a description of any findings, diagnosis and treatment, final disposition of the patient (including instructions given), and the condition of the patient on discharge or transfer.

The record is to be signed by the physician in attendance. A control register should be kept. The emergency room medical records should be used to regularly evaluate the quality of emergency medical care.

In 1978 JCAH upgraded its emergency services standards.[2] The new standards classify emergency rooms by four levels of care, characterized as Levels I through IV. Level I, expected to be satisfied nationwide by no more than 40 large teaching hospitals, requires qualifying medical facilities to provide comprehensive round-the-clock coverage by at least one physically present, on-duty physician who is experienced in the treatment of emergency patients, as well as in-house physician coverage for several specialty services. Like Level I, Level II requires 24-hour service by an on-duty emergency care physician, although at this level specialty consultation need only be available within 30 minutes. Level III, expected to apply to the largest single group of hospitals, requires 24-hour coverage by a physician not necessarily experienced in emergency care. Finally, the Level IV hospital emergency room is required merely to determine whether an emergency exists, to render life-saving first aid, and to transfer the patient to the nearest appropriate institution.

Irrespective of the level of care, the new standards require that emergency room head nurses be qualified by "relevant training, experience, and current competence." Added provisions require that Level I, II, and III facilities have "readily available at all times clinical laboratory services . . . [capable] of performing all . . . standard [body specimen] analyses." Prior JCAH guidelines mandated that hospital emergency rooms maintain a "control register" recording the name, date, and time of arrival of "each patient served." The revised standards also require that hospitals record the nature of the patient's complaint, its disposition, and the time of the patient's departure "for every individual seeking care." In addition, there must now be formal training programs for emergency care personnel. The standards further require that the emergency services director conduct monthly quality control reviews to assure quality patient care.

Although JCAH standards are neither laws nor regulations, hospitals voluntarily ascribe to these standards for the purpose of accreditation. Additionally, these standards establish Medicare eligibility. Legally, these standards can be used in a court of law to show adherence or lack of adherence on the part of a hospital that is a party to the suit, as they were in *Guerrero* v. *Copper Queen Hospital,* 22 Ariz. App. 611, 529 P.2d 1205, rehearing denied 531 P.2d 548 (1975).

LIABILITY IN GENERAL

In addition to the legal right to function, there is the legal issue of liability. Administrators and health care professionals need to understand this issue and their rights and obligations under the law. The rest of this chapter will deal with the issue of liability including strict liability in tort, the elements of a negligence action, vicarious liability, and issues involved in statutes of limitation.

In the case of a hospital, as well as for professionals, the law looks to whether the standard of care owed to patients, visitors, staff, and employees has been breached. The courts have traditionally held that any hospital, as well as any practitioner, owes patients that degree of care, skill, and diligence generally exercised by hospitals and practitioners in the same locality. Recently this narrow rule has been broadened by some courts to mean the degree of care, skill, and diligence exercised by hospitals or practitioners in similar (as opposed to the same) localities. This broader rule makes it possible to establish liability in a greater number of cases than under the narrower rule.

The broader rule has come into recent prominence because of the easier access to information and knowledge of good standards of practice. With present improvements in travel, communication, and media, there is little justification for ignorance or lack of knowledge of good practice techniques. Thus courts are increasingly willing to use the broader rule, which could lead to a finding of liability the narrower rule would have precluded. In a court using the broader rule, a hospital or a health professional would not be allowed to defend against an action for negligence by claiming adherence to the practice of others in the same locality.

Strict Liability

Strict liability is absolute liability or liability without fault. A case is one of strict liability when neither care nor negligence, neither good nor bad faith, neither knowledge nor ignorance will save the defendant.

One may not be negligent, but liability may be imposed by statute. This is rare in health law, where the instances of liability overwhelmingly involve issues of negligence. Strict liability is a matter of public policy, and in the area of health care these cases most often involve blood transfusions. Here the courts have had to distinguish whether blood was a product sold or a service rendered to the patient. The distinction becomes important because if the blood is deemed to have been sold, and if the patient was harmed by adulterated or infected blood, strict liability in tort —that is, liability without fault— may apply. In *Brody* v. *Overlook Hospital,* 66 N.J. 448, 332 A. 2d 596 (1975), the court held that in this case, arising before new testing methods were available, the plaintiff had to prove that the blood infection with hepatitis was caused by the negligence of either the hospital or the blood bank before damages could be recovered. The availability of new testing may make hospitals and blood banks strictly liable for defective blood in the future.

Similarly, in *Cunningham* v. *MacNeal Memorial Hospital,* 113 Ill. App. 2d 74 251 N.E. 2d 773, modified, 47 Ill. 2d 443, 266 N.E. 2d 897 (1970), the plaintiff appealed a judgment in favor of the defendant hospital. The lower court had felt that the plaintiff had erroneously stated a cause of action "against this defendant upon the theory that blood is a product, that such product was furnished in a defective and unreasonably dangerous condition and that by reason thereof defendant is strictly liable to plaintiff for her alleged damages." The appellate court reversed and remanded the case, holding that the plaintiff had stated a cause of action and was entitled to try to prove her case. As to the issue of the sale of blood as a product, the court said:

> It would appear that the real reason some would refrain from calling human blood a product is the belief that those dealing in it are doctors, hospitals and blood banks, who perform a meritorious service for the community and are entitled to preferential treatment from the law. However, our Supreme Court has indicated that a hospital should not be treated any differently from any other organization; . . .

> In the instant case the defendant argues that blood cannot properly be classified as a product. In this connection we note that a Federal Trade Commission opinion was handed down in June 1964. . . . The synopsis of the opinion noted that the examiner had rejected various "jurisdictional issues," among them the claim that human blood was not subject to F.T.C. control because blood was not an article of commerce. The synopsis . . . concluded that blood is subject to trade and commerce within the meaning of the terms as used in the F.T.C. Act. . . .

> *   *   *

> We believe it is realistic and reasonable to hold that a sale is involved in the transaction whereby the patient comes into possession of blood. On oral argument in the case before us counsel for the hospital stated that a sale was not involved; that rather, there was an exchange of personal property for remuneration. That is an attempt to make a distinction without a difference . . .
>
> *Cunningham* v. *MacNeal Memorial Hospital,*
> 251 N.E. 2d at 735 ff.

The Illinois Supreme Court agreed with the appellate court and thus held that the plaintiff had stated a strict liability cause of action against the hospital. The court felt that this was more fair than permitting such a loss to fall on an individual consumer who was entirely without fault in the matter. This was despite the fact that there was no way to detect the existence of serum hepatitis virus in the blood.

As stated earlier, strict liability in tort is rarely seen in health care law, and when it is seen it usually involves product liability, the product usually being blood. For the most part, liability for hospitals and health care professionals is an issue of negligence.

Negligence

The vast majority of litigation against hospitals, nurses, and physicians is based on claims of negligence. This section will deal with the principles of negligence and the application of these principles by the courts.

A hospital may be found liable for the negligence of others under the doctrine of respondeat superior. It may also be found liable for its own negligence in not observing a standard of care to a patient or others. This is termed corporate negligence. Liability for hospitals is predicated on issues of defective and improper equipment, the physical condition of the premises, and negligent drug handling. It can also be predicated on medical treatment.

Negligence by nurses and physicians is termed malpractice. The courts use the standard of conduct of liability for professionals to determine what is or is not negligent practice. Simply put, malpractice is professional negligence. An action for malpractice is a tort action and thus is part of the civil, as opposed to the criminal, law.

Prior to the well publicized leading case of *Darling* v. *Charleston Community Memorial Hospital,* 33 Ill. 2d 326, 211 N.E. 2d 253 (1965), cert. denied, 383 U.S. 946 (1966), hospitals in the United States generally enjoyed charitable immunity from suit. The doctrine of charitable immunity was first applied in a Massachusetts court a century ago to protect hospitals against loss of assets that might be diminished by lawsuits. It was reasoned that the loss of assets for charitable purposes was contrary to public policy. Until the *Darling* case, the reasoning was generally followed by U.S. state courts. However, the doctrine has generally been abandoned in the United States in recognition of the belief that charitable institutions, like businesses, should compensate people for the injuries they cause. It has also been noted that charitable institutions can purchase liability insurance for protection.

The *Darling* case did hold the hospital liable for harm to a patient that resulted from the improper application of a leg cast. Although the patient complained repeatedly of pain and his toes became swollen and dark in color, proper treatment was not instituted and eventually amputation was necessary. The court held that the hospital's liability under the concept of corporate neglect or under respondeat superior was adequately supported by either of the two allegations urged by the plaintiff:

> [That the hospital had] failed to have a sufficient number of trained nurses for bedside care of all patients at all times capable of recognizing the progressive gangrenous condition of the plaintiff's right leg, and of bringing the same to the attention of the hospital administration and to the medical staff so that adequate consultation could have been secured and such conditions rectified; . . . [and] [f]ailed to require consultation with or examination by members of the hospital surgical staff skilled in such treatment; or to review the treatment rendered to the plaintiff and to require consultants to be called in as needed.
>
> *Darling* v. *Charleston Community Memorial Hospital,* 211 N.E. 2d 253 at 258.

Using a similar rationale, the court in *Pederson* v. *Dumochel,* 72 Wash. 2d 73, 431 P. 2d 973 (1967), held a hospital liable for injury caused when the patient suffered oxygen deprivation of the brain while undergoing dental surgery. In *Pederson* the hospital broke its own rule in not requiring the presence of a physician during the dental surgery.

Likewise, where a plaintiff's decedent died from the effects of a strep throat after childbirth, the hospital breached the standard of care embodied in its own documents. The liability for a patient's death, in *Foley* v. *Bishop Clarkson Memorial Hospital,* 173 N.W. 2d 881 (Nebr. 1970), was held to be a jury question. The defendant hospital failed to obey its rules requiring that a history and results of a physical examination be written within 24 hours after the patient's admission, and that personnel were to observe the patient closely and report suspected infections, hemorrhage, change of blood pressure or pulse, and other symptoms of complications to the attending physician. This was permitted to be used as evidence of negligence before a jury, and together with other evidence, was to be used to show the standard of care prevalent in Omaha or similar communities. The court held that a jury question was presented as to whether the hospital adhered to community standards. Thus a new trial was ordered.

Other courts have construed the *Darling* decision as a possible basis for imposing liability on a hospital for imprudent or careless selection of staff members, for example in *Mauer* v. *Highland Park Hospital Foundation,* 90 Ill. App. 2d 409, 232 N.E. 2d 776 (1967). For further recognition of the hospital's responsibility to exercise due care in the selection of physicians as members of the medical staff, see *Joiner* v. *Mitchell County Hospital,* 186 S.E. 2d 307 (1971).

Adherence to institutional and departmental policies is an essential protection against hospital liability. To avoid liability, it is vital that a hospital consistently practice accepted standards of conduct and adhere to accepted institutional and departmental policies. Courts will look to evidence of prudent practice to determine whether or not liability attaches. For a fuller treatment of this topic see Chapter 10 (*Yeargin et al.* v. *Hamilton Memorial Hospital*) and Chapter 3 (*Niles* v. *City of San Rafael*).

In addition to the corporate negligence of an institution, a hospital also may be found liable for the negligence of its employees under the doctrine of respondeat superior, a form of vicarious liability. Vicarious liability will be discussed following a general discussion of malpractice and negligence.

Malpractice

In law, liability for malpractice is predicated on negligent behavior. In this tort action, one party alleges or claims that wrongful conduct on the part of the professional nurse or physician has caused harm. Compensation is sought for the harm suffered. In order to establish that professional behavior or conduct was negligent, four elements must be proved in a court of law. The first element is duty. Health professionals have a legal duty to protect patients against unreasonable risks of harm. Second, it must be proved that a breach of duty occurred. The third element is causation. It is imperative that a connection be shown between the health professional's conduct and the alleged harm. The fourth element is damages or the harm itself. In order to be awarded damages in court, the plaintiff must show personal injury. Personal injury can consist of economic loss, actual injury (which could be physical, psychological, or both), and pain and suffering. The presence of the first three elements without the fourth would constitute an incomplete tort action and would fail. All four elements must be present.

Duty and Breach of Duty

For the first two elements, the legal standard of conduct and care is that of the reasonably prudent professional. If the defendant were a nurse, the standard would be that of a reasonably prudent nurse. If the defendant were a physician, the standard would be that of a reasonably prudent physician. Thus, in the case of a physician, malpractice would consist of failing to do what a reasonably prudent physician would have done or having done what a reasonably prudent physician would not have done in a specific situation.

To determine whether a professional nurse or physician has been negligent, the court or jury must decide what the reasonably prudent nurse or physician would have done in the same or a similar situation. The nurse or physician is then held to that level of performance.

Because the judge or jury is not trained or qualified to determine the standard of care of the reasonably prudent nurse or physician, to establish this level of performance the courts generally rely on the services of expert witnesses. These are persons who are trained in nursing or medicine and who can testify as to the professional standard of care in the same or similar communities. An expert witness must be of the same profession as the defendant; a nurse cannot serve as an expert witness in medicine, and a physician cannot serve as an expert witness in nursing. The testimony of the expert provides the standard by which the actual conduct of the nurse or physician is measured. If the actual conduct falls below the standard established, the nurse or physician will be found to have been negligent.

Expert witnesses are considered necessary in the vast majority of malpractice cases. However, expert witnesses will not be necessary in a case where the court or jury can clearly see that negligence occurred. In one court case,. *Thomas* v. *Corso,* 228 A. 2d 37 (Ct. App. Md., 1972), a physician was charged with malpractice for not rendering emergency care to a man who had been hit by a car. The court found that expert testimony was not necessary because the ordinary person could readily understand the damage that could be done to a human body by an automobile and could understand the physician was negligent in not examining the patient.

The ability to foresee the consequences of professional conduct is one concept courts consider in determining the standard of conduct. Two Canadian cases show how the courts apply foreseeability to the elements of duty and breach of duty. In the first case, the nurse-defendant was held negligent. In the second case, negligence was not found.

In the first case, a patient suffered permanent brain damage as the result of receiving insufficient oxygen while in a recovery room following the administration of anesthesia during surgery. The problem resulted because the one nurse on duty had too little time to care for the patient properly. Two persons were found negligent: a second nurse who had been on a coffee break, and the supervisor who authorized her absence. As an expert witness for the plaintiff, a nursing supervisor testified that normally two nurses were present in the recovery room and that both nurses were expected to take their coffee breaks before any patients arrived from the operating room. When the one nurse left for a coffee break, two patients had already been admitted to the recovery room. The court held, in *Laidlaw* v. *Lion's Gate Hospital,* 70 Western Weekly Reports 729 (1969), that the supervisor as well as the nurse knew the operating room schedule and thus should have foreseen that the two nurses were needed on duty.

In the second Canadian case, negligence was not established. In *Child* v. *Vancouver General Hospital and Tennessy,* 71 Western Weekly Reports 648 (1970), the nurse had left a patient unattended while she took a coffee break because a physician had just seen the patient and the patient seemed much improved. The court held that the nurse could not have foreseen an increased risk to the patient if she left for a coffee break.

It must be clearly understood that in a negligence action, the plaintiff must prove that the defendant owed the plaintiff a duty of reasonable care. In order to determine whether a duty in fact exists, the court examines the relationship between the parties. The duty of a nurse or physician to a patient arises when the professional voluntarily enters into a health care relationship with the patient. If it were not for this voluntary assumption of a health care relationship, there would be no duty on the part of the professional and the suit would fail for lack of the element of duty. In the law, in general, the bystander has no duty to render aid to an injured person, whether or not that bystander is a health care professional. Thus, the issue of relationship is crucial.

It is important that emergency room personnel recognize the growing acknowledgment of courts that hospitals have a duty to patients to provide emergency care when it is requested. Under the common law, neither the physician nor the private hospital had a duty to render medical treatment. As a result it was possible for hospitals to refuse to render emergency treatment to individuals who requested it. But this situation has been reversed as a result of a series of legal decisions that grew out of abuses in emergency departments of general hospitals. The hospital's right to refuse emergency service to a patient has subsequently been substantially curtailed. This reversal and the growing trend toward recognizing the hospital's duty to provide emergency care began with a Delaware case, *Wilmington General Hospital* v. *Manlove,* 54 Del. 15, 174 A. 2d 135 (1961). *Manlove* was based on the issue of reliance, that is, the community's reliance on an emergency room that existed to provide necessary emergency care. This case will be dealt with comprehensively in Chapter 3.

Causation

The third element in an action for professional negligence or malpractice is causation. Causation is important because even though a duty and a breach of duty may be established, unless that breach of duty is shown to be the cause of the patient's injury, liability will not attach.

In these days of talk about the practice of defensive medicine and defensive nursing, one may be tempted to think that every slight breach of duty results in litigation. This is far from the truth. In fact, there may be many more instances of breach of duty that never result in lawsuits. This is because every situation in which a breach of duty occurs does not result in or cause an injury.

For example, suppose a physician means to prescribe a certain dose of medication for a patient. Consider further that the medication is prescribed to induce sleep. Negligently, the physician prescribes half the dose intended. If this error in dosage causes no injury to the patient, then no liability will attach. What if the patient then slipped and fell on a wet floor and suffered injury? It would be difficult if not impossible to connect this injury to the too-small dosage of medication.

It is often extremely difficult to prove causation. This is because there may be variable causes for an injury, and it is often difficult to clearly identify a connection between negligent conduct and a later injury. In addition, the courts look for proximate cause. Proximate cause is that which, in a natural and continuous sequence, unbroken by any efficient intervening cause, produces the injury, and without which the result would not have occurred.

In *McBride* v. *United States,* 462 Fed. 2d 72 (9th Cir., 1972), the issue was proximate cause. Suit was brought by the widow of a retired naval officer who had died of a heart attack. The plaintiff alleged that her husband's death was proximately caused by the negligent failure of the army hospital doctor to admit her husband to a coronary care unit. The case was dismissed during the course of the trial because the plaintiff had not established the requisite causal proximity between the lack of hospital treatment and the patient's death.

The facts of the case revealed that the decedent had previously spent five days in the hospital coronary ward undergoing tests to diagnose the source of pain in his lower chest. The tests revealed no evidence of heart disease. The decedent was released and asked to return in a few weeks for further testing. Three nights after discharge, the decedent again experienced severe chest pains. He presented himself at the emergency room of the defendant hospital. The resident on duty examined him, read the report of the earlier testing, and took an electrocardiogram. By this time the decedent's pain had subsided and his vital signs were normal. The resident told the decedent that his chest pain probably resulted from a gastrointestinal disturbance, but that heart disease could not be ruled out. He advised admission to the coronary care unit. The decedent preferred to return home, stating that he felt fine and that previous hospitalization had disclosed no problems with his heart. The physician allowed him to return home on condition that he return at once should the pain recur. The patient died shortly after reaching home.

The plaintiff sought to prove that the doctor on duty had been negligent in his diagnosis and should have insisted the patient be hospitalized. The appellate court ruled that the plaintiff's evidence showing that the decedent would have a significantly greater chance (50 percent greater) of surviving a heart attack if treated in a coronary care unit was enough to show that it was a reasonable medical probability. Because nonadmittance could be causally connected to the patient's death, the case was reversed and remanded for a new trial. Plaintiff would not need to prove with certainty that the injury would not have occurred after proper treatment, since the best medical treatment in the world could not provide an absolute guarantee of success. For another example of how courts view the element of duty, see *Nance* v. *James Archer Smith Hospital, Inc.*, discussed fully in Chapter 5.

In *Thomas* v. *Corso*, 265 Md. 84, 288 A. 2d 379 (1972), the issues of cause and proximate cause were important to the resolution of the case. The facts in this case reveal that Corso was hit by a car while he was standing on the highway. He was taken to the emergency room of the nearest hospital. Although the on-call physician was called approximately 15 minutes after the plaintiff was admitted to the emergency room, he did not come to examine the patient until some three hours later and pronounced the patient dead when he (the doctor) arrived at the hospital.

The physician was found guilty of malpractice for failure to attend to the patient because common sense would indicate that without attention the consequences of a human body being hit by an automobile could be serious, and that failure to attend the decedent did not meet standards of reasonable care.

But the defendant-physician contended that the plaintiff failed to establish the causal connection between his alleged negligence and Corso's death. The court disagreed with this contention, saying:

> Dr. Thomas' admission that he believed he might have helped Corso, might have revived Corso if he had been called at 12:05 a.m. and that lack of treatment by a physician increased Corso's danger of losing his life . . . [was] sufficient to justify a jury finding of a substantial possibility of survival which was destroyed by the failure of Dr. Thomas to examine, diagnose and treat Corso at any time after Corso arrived at the Emergency Room and was accepted by Dr. Thomas as his patient.

> Dr. Thomas also contends that if it be assumed that he was negligent, there must exist not only a causal connection between the negligence complained of and the injury suffered, but further that the connection must be by a natural and unbroken sequence—without intervening efficient causes—so that but for the negligence of the defendant, the injury would not have occurred. The defendant's negligence must not only be a cause but must be a proximate cause of the injury . . . Dr. Thomas urges that the proximate cause of Corso's death was either the intervening cause of the negligence of the on-duty nurses

or the inevitability of death due to the nature of Corso's injuries. He contends that his "uncontradicted" testimony establishes this. We do not see it that way . . .

From what we have already stated, the jury could have reasonably concluded that under the circumstances of this case that if Dr. Thomas had performed his duty to attend Corso personally shortly after he was telephoned at 11:30 p.m., Dr. Thomas might well have been able to have saved his life and that this negligent conduct was one of the direct and proximate causes of Corso's death, concurrent with the negligence of the nurses.

Thomas v. *Corso,* 288 A. 2d 379 at 390.

In *Cooper* v. *Sisters of Charity of Cincinnati,* 27 Ohio St. 2d 242, 272 N.E. 2d 97 (1971) (Sup. Ct. Ohio, 1971), actual and proximate cause were not established and liability did not attach. The facts in *Cooper* revealed that a 16-year-old boy was struck by a truck while riding his bicycle. He was taken to the emergency room of Good Samaritan Hospital where a physician examined him. Although the boy had been hit on the back of his head, the examining physician did not examine that area. The boy was discharged after the examination. He was to be observed closely at home and returned to the emergency room if necessary. The boy remained awake with no apparent change in his condition, until becoming restless just before his death, which occurred early the next morning. An autopsy determined that the cause of death was a basal skull fracture—the result of an injury to his head, and a swelling of the tissues in the back of the head, causing intracranial pressure and hemorrhage.

Expert testimony was elicited to state that there was practically a 100 percent mortality rate without surgery for patients with similar injuries, and that there was "maybe some place around 50 percent" chance that the decedent would have survived with the surgery.

The appellate court affirmed the judgment of the lower court in favor of the defendants, citing the trial judge's conclusions of law as follows:

From the facts adduced it is the conclusion of the court that the evidence of proximate cause was insufficient to make a prima facie case for submission to the jury as against defendant . . .

Reasonable minds could arrive at differing conclusions as to whether Dr. Hansen was negligent in rendering professional medical services to plaintiff's decedent, and there is sufficient evidence for the submission of that issue to the jury . . .

The more problematic issue of proximate cause looms from these facts . . .

It has been established, and we now reaffirm the principle that: "Even though there is evidence of malpractice sufficient for submission to the jury on that issue, a verdict must be directed in favor of the defendant where there is no evidence adduced which would give rise to a reasonable inference that the defendant's acts (sic) of malpractice was the direct and proximate cause of the injury to the plaintiff."

*   *   *

In an action for wrongful death, where medical malpractice is alleged as the proximate cause of death, and plaintiff's evidence indicates that a failure to diagnose the injury prevented the patient from an opportunity to be operated on, which failure eliminated any chance of the patient's survival, the issue of proximate cause can be submitted to a jury only if there is sufficient evidence showing that with proper diagnosis, treatment and surgery the patient probably would have survived.

Cooper v. *Sisters of Charity of Cincinnati, Inc.,* 272 N.E. 2d 97 at 102 and 104.

Because the plaintiff was unable to produce this evidence, proximate cause was not established and judgment was rendered for the defendants. The court felt that "maybe" and "around" 50 percent did not connote a medical probability (as was found in *McBride*). Those words could mean either more than 50 percent or less than 50 percent, and the court held that "(p)robable is *more* than 50 percent of actual," *Cooper,* 272 N.E. 2d 97 at 104. Thus proximate cause was not established since the probability of survival with the surgery was not proved by the plaintiff. In every case each one of the four elements of negligence must be proved by a preponderance of the evidence, which in percentage terms would be 51 percent or greater.

Damages

The fourth element necessary for a successful tort action is that of damages or actual injury. This is a crucial factor because if the suit cannot prove actual harm it will be unsuccessful. For example, imagine a breach of duty in which harmless vitamins are given to the wrong patient. In this situation there has clearly been a negligent act, but because no harm or injury results, no legal action can be brought.

It is essential to remember that in negligence actions, the aim is not to impose a fine and penalty as in criminal law, but to assess money damages to compensate the victim for the injury suffered. Thus where there is no injury, there can be no compensation. The plaintiff must prove that he or she incurred damages as a result of the alleged negligence. If the plaintiff has not incurred damages, suit will not be successful.

In *Niles* v. *City of San Rafael,* 42 Cal. App. 230, 116 Cal. Rptr. 733 (1974), the jury awarded plaintiffs $4,025,000. In *Niles* the plaintiffs brought a negligence action against a city, its school district, a hospital, and the director of the hospital's pediatric outpatient clinic for permanent injury to an 11-year-old boy as a result of inadequate emergency care following a schoolyard injury. Due to a variety of errors, the boy was discharged prematurely and suffered intracranial bleeding. Although surgery was performed successfully to remove a blood clot, it was too late to prevent permanent, irreparable brain damage. His condition would never be able to be improved by medical or surgical treatment. The child was left totally disabled; except for slight movements of the right hand and foot, he was paralyzed from the neck down. He was mute, although he could communicate by eye movements and could hear and see well. Although his body was paralyzed, his mental capacities appeared to be unaffected.

At the trial the jury found the city and the school district negligent in the supervision of the playground. The medical defendants were found to have committed professional malpractice. Under California law of proximate causation, the city and the school district were liable for all of plaintiff's damages. The medical defendants were jointly liable with the city and school district for the damages caused by the malpractice. However, the common law of California also provides for the second tort feasors, under these circumstances, to assume that portion of the damages directly attributable to them. In other words the medical defendants (or second tort feasors) had to indemnify the city and school district for the damages that the medical defendants caused. Under this rule the jury allocated $25,000 to the public entities and $4,000,000 to the medical defendants.

Damages, as a rule, are impossible to fix with any certainty. It is important to remember however that in a tort action the purpose of damages is to make the injured party whole again, to restore the injured party to his or her original position. In general, tort damages consist of nominal damages, compensatory damages, and punitive damages. In most tort actions the most important of these is compensatory damages. This is because an injured plaintiff has the right of recovery for all the damage caused by the negligent act, whether or not the results were to be reasonably anticipated.

As to the issue of excessive judgment, the rule is that an appellate court may not interfere with an award unless "the verdict is so large that, at first blush, it shocks the conscience and suggests passion, prejudice, or corruption on the part of the jury," *Seffert* v. *Los Angeles Transit Lines,* 15 Cal. Rptr. 161, 166 as quoted in *Niles* v. *City of San Rafael,* 116 Cal. Rptr. 733, 739.

The plaintiffs introduced evidence at trial to support the following composition of the verdict:

Lost earnings	$503,570.
Past medical expenses	86,240.
Future medical expenses	196,902.
Cost of medical supplies and equipment	41,637.
Medical emergency fund	50,000.
Tutoring and instruction	242,643.
Attendant care	1,299,637.
Total economic loss	$2,420,629.
General Damages	1,604,371.
Total	$4,025,000.

Each item of future expense was supported by expert testimony covering the boy's life expectancy, the current cost of the various services, estimates of future inflation, and U.S. Labor Department studies. The present value of the future expenses was calculated by a five percent discount rate. This figure was supported by commercial investment studies, Federal Reserve System studies, and statistics from the United States Savings and Loan League.

General damages are to compensate for pain, fright, grief, humiliation, embarrassment, anxiety, and other associated mental injuries. In view of the boy's condition the court was not prepared to say that the award of approximately $1.6 million was excessive.

In *Niles* the plaintiffs were able to sustain their claims of damage by expert testimony. They were thus able to recover general damages for pain and suffering and special damages for loss of earnings, health care costs, tutoring and instruction.

Res Ipsa Loquitur

Heretofore, we have discussed the four elements that must be proved in a successful suit for negligence. One of the elements—causation—is essential to show the relationship or connection between the harm or injury suffered and the negligence (by act or omission) of the person alleged to be responsible.

The doctrine of res ipsa loquitur, a Latin phrase meaning "the thing speaks for itself," exists to assist plaintiffs in recovering damages in situations where it would be virtually impossible to prove all the elements of negligence. In order to raise res ipsa loquitur, plaintiffs need to prove: (1) that the injury or harm suffered does not ordinarily occur in the absence of negligence, (2) that the harm or injury resulted from an instrument in the exclusive control of the defendant, and (3) that the patient could not have voluntarily contributed to his or her own injury.

In medical malpractice cases, res ipsa loquitur is most often raised in cases involving surgery with the patient anesthetized and therefore unaware of how the injury occurred. The classic res ipsa loquitur situation would involve a patient who undergoes surgery for an inflamed appendix and awakes from anesthesia with a sharp pain in his or her leg. It would be extremely difficult, if not impossible, for the plaintiff to prove negligence because the anesthetic precluded alertness during the time the injury occurred. *Ybarra* v. *Spangard* 25 Cal. 2d 486, 154 P.2d 687 (1944).

Ordinarily a plaintiff in a negligence case must prove the acts that constitute the defendant's negligence. The doctrine of res ipsa loquitur allows the plaintiff to reach the jury even though he or she can produce no direct proof that these acts occurred.

In *Davis* v. *Memorial Hospital*, 58 Cal. 2d 815, 26 Cal. Rptr. 633, 376 P. 2d 561 (1962), the Supreme Court of California recognized that the doctrine of res ipsa loquitur may be conditionally employed. In this case, the plaintiff entered the defendant hospital for a varicose vein operation and was given a presurgical enema. Although the operation was successful, the defendant thereafter developed a perirectal abscess necessitating several weeks of treatment. Surgery was later required to close a fistula resulting from the abscess. The trial court refused plaintiff an instruction on res ipsa loquitur for the reason that there was conflicting testimony as to whether the abscess was caused by the administration of the enema. The Supreme Court of California reversed the trial court, holding that since there was conflicting evidence as to whether the administration of the enema caused the abscess, the plaintiff was entitled to have the judge explain the applicability and the doctrine of res ipsa loquitur to the jury. However, in *Clemens* v. *Regents of University of California,* 87 Cal. Rptr. 108, 8 Cal. App. 3d 1 (1970), a California District Court of Appeals refused to sanction a conditional res ipsa loquitur instruction for the reason that the medical procedure involved was highly complex, and the harm therefore gave rise to no presumption of negligence in the performance of the procedure.

In *Edgar County Bank and Trust Co.* v. *Paris Hospital, Inc.,* 57 Ill. 2d 298, 312 N.E. 2d 259 (1974), the court found that the doctrine of res ipsa loquitur stated a cause of action in a situation arising from emergency care. The patient—a 17-month-old child—suffered permanent injuries, including foot drop and permanent impairment of the foot and calf, from a hypodermic needle negligently inserted by a hospital emergency room physician. The plaintiff claimed he had no control over the injection, that it had been in the exclusive control of the hospital and its employees. The court said that res ipsa loquitur was appropriate in a case such as this where the direct evidence of the cause of the injury was in control of the defendant. The doctrine is accepted and applied by all of the courts, including those of South Carolina (which purports to reject it by name), Michigan (which formerly did so), and Pennsylvania (which purports to limit its application to cases in which the defendant has voluntarily undertaken some responsibility).[3]

However, a large number of states do not allow that the doctrine of res ipsa loquitur is applicable in cases of medical or hospital malpractice. This, combined with the fact that it appears that the doctrine is used infrequently in emergency care cases, suggests that it is not a matter of burning urgency to staff members of emergency departments of general hospitals.

Vicarious Liability

It is important that health professionals and administrators understand the concept of vicarious liability. Respondeat superior is a form of vicarious liability whereby an employer is held liable for the negligent behavior of employees.

The fact situation is extremely important in each case to determine where liability lies and if respondeat superior applies. Respondeat superior or "let the master answer" is the phrase used to express the area of the master's liability for torts of servants arising out of service to the master. The rationale for the doctrine is twofold: first, the master should pay for torts committed by servants in return for the benefits the master receives from the servant's proper conduct; and second, the master is better able than the servant to sustain the loss through insurance or other means.

In order for liability to attach under the doctrine of respondeat superior, the plaintiff must show that the negligent behavior occurred within the scope of the employee's employment and that a master-servant relationship existed between employer and employee. To prove scope of employment, the plaintiff needs to show that the act is closely related to what the employee was hired to do. To prove the master-servant relationship, the plaintiff must show that the employer had control over the physical actions of the employee in the performance of assigned duties. The doctrine of respondeat superior does not apply in the case of independent contractors. Thus attending physicians and private duty nurses are not generally covered by this doctrine.

Even when respondeat superior applies, it does not render the defendant-employee immune from suit. Professionals are always independently liable for their own negligent behavior.

Legally, if the employer must compensate an injured party for the employee's negligence, the employer may then seek indemnification from that employee. Indemnification allows the employer to recover the financial loss from the negligent employee.

Within the emergency room setting, it is important to understand the law of agency. The law of agency includes every relation in which one person acts for or represents another by the latter's authority. This covers the relationships of principal and agent, master and servant, or employer/proprietor and independent contractor.

It is important to determine the exact relationship in order to ascertain liability correctly. Obviously, because of the variety of relationships in the typical emergency room setting, liability may fall totally on one party or may be shared among a number of parties. Emergency department staff members must remember that from a legal standpoint individuals are responsible for their own torts, irrespective of whether they are independent contractors or hospital employees. Generally, an employee's negligence, if committed within the scope of employment, renders the employer vicariously liable under the legal rule of agency. However, in general the torts of an independent contractor are not vicariously imputed to the employer if the employer does not significantly control the actions of the independent contractor.

The law of agency, in distributing liability, sounds a lot simpler than it actually is. It is not enough to say that an employer is vicariously liable for the negligent behavior of an employee. The individual facts of each case must be analyzed carefully to determine the exact relationship that exists. The facts of the case may create variations within the general law.

Once they understand the notion of agency law, emergency department staff members may be better able to understand why plaintiffs attempt to join each and every possible defendant in an action for negligence in their attempts to recover damages or be compensated by whomever the court determines is the liable party. It should also be noted that when an action for negligence is brought against the hospital and individual professional staff members, each side will try to demonstrate that liability clearly rests with the other party.

When a patient brings suit against emergency department staff members for not rendering services according to the appropriate standards of care, that patient can choose to sue in tort or for breach of contract. Because recovery is almost always much higher in tort than in contract, and for other reasons, more cases will be brought as negligence actions than for breach of contract.

Under tort law, the hospital's liability can be predicated on a theory of corporate negligence or on respondeat superior. We have already seen the theory of corporate negligence applied in *Darling* v. *Charleston Community Memorial Hospital,* 33 Ill. 2d 326, 211 N.E. 2d 253 (1965), cert. denied, 383 U.S. 946 (1966). However, it must be remembered that the court was willing to find the defendant hospital liable under the theory of corporate negligence or the theory of respondeat superior for the negligence of the hospital employees. The theory of corporate negligence was emphasized in *Darling* on the basis of the hospital's duty as defined in accreditation rules and the hospital's own by-laws as a way to do away with the doctrine of charitable immunity for hospitals.

Hospitals have been able to avoid liability for the negligence of their employees under the doctrine of respondeat superior by raising the defense that the employee was an independent contractor or borrowed servant. Hospitals have had varying degrees of success with these defenses. As mentioned before, the facts of each individual case have been extremely important in ascertaining where liability is fixed.

Stated once again, respondeat superior is a form of vicarious liability whereby an employer is held liable for the wrongful acts of an employee even though the employer's conduct is without fault. Hence, it is substituted liability. Before liability predicated on respondeat superior may be imposed on an employer, it is necessary that the plaintiff prove a master-servant relationship did exist between the employer and employee, and that the wrongful act occurred within the scope of that person's employment. The test for determining whether a master-servant relationship exists is whether the employer has the right to control the physical conduct of the employee in the performance of his or her duties. An act is within the scope of employment if the act is so closely related to what the employee has been hired to do, or so fairly and reasonably incidental to his or her employment, that it may be regarded as a method, although improper, of carrying out the orders of the employer. There are a multiplicity of factors that a court would invariably consider in order to determine whether a relationship is defined as employment or independent contractor, including method of compensation, ownership of equipment, existence of fringe benefits, and the intent of the parties. (See Chapter 10 for an elaboration of this concept.)

The doctrine of respondeat superior does not absolve the employee of liability for the wrongful act. The injured party may sue the employee directly. In addition, the employer may seek indemnification from the employee. Because the employee is primarily responsible for the loss, the law does not relieve him or her of liability in cases where the hospital is held liable through the application of respondeat superior.

The doctrine of respondeat superior does not apply in the instance of wrongful conduct by an independent contractor. In the case of an independent contractor, the principal usually has no right of control over the manner in which the work is performed. This lack of the right of control makes the enterprise that of the independent contractor, rather than that of the employer.

Originally the doctrine of respondeat superior only applied to the negligent acts of an employee. The trend of court decisions, however, seems to be one of broadening substantially the meaning of "scope of employment" to include within its coverage personal failings of the employee which have some causal relationship to his employment.

The "borrowed servant" doctrine may apply under respondeat superior in certain fact situations to impose liability upon a physician or surgeon rather than upon the hospital. Currently the trend is away from finding liability under this doctrine.

A hospital is generally not liable for the wrongful conduct of a staff physician or surgeon who treats patients in the hospital. Most often emphasis is placed on the contract for medical treatment between patient and physician and on the fact that the hospital has no right to control the physician's conduct in administering to the patient. Although this situation does occasionally arise in the context of an emergency room setting, more often the court needs to distinguish between the physician employed by the hospital to staff the emergency room and the physician employed by the hospital as an independent contractor whose job it is to staff the emergency room.

Some courts have begun to propound the theory of ostensible or apparent agency to impose respondeat superior liability upon hospitals. In these cases the courts have held that it was up to the jury to determine whether the physician involved was an employee or an independent contractor.

Hospitals have been held liable under respondeat superior for the wrongful acts of residents, interns, and nurses. Basically, these three categories of hospital employees are treated similarly in cases where respondeat superior applies. Residents, interns, or nurses may, by their wrongful conduct, subject a hospital to liability under respondeat superior. On the other hand, each of them may become the "borrowed servant" of a staff physician or surgeon, and liability for their tortious conduct will therefore rest with the physician or surgeon. (As mentioned earlier, the "borrowed servant" doctrine is not as popular now as it was in earlier decades.)

A resident is one who pursues a course of advanced medical study in a hospital, under the direction of a staff physician or department. In addition, the resident is paid a salary by the hospital to perform certain routine duties. There is no contractual relationship between the resident and the patients whom he or she treats. The absence of such a contractual relationship, and the fact that the resident is a salaried employee of the hospital, generally leads courts to apply the doctrine of respondeat superior and impose liability upon the hospital, without giving much consideration to the hospital's right to control its residents. Even though a resident is to some extent under the supervision of a staff physician, when the resident performs those functions for which he or she was hired by the hospital, the hospital is liable for the resident's wrongful conduct under the doctrine of respondeat superior. In cases where the resident is under the direction of a department head employed by the hospital, there is no question but that respondeat superior would apply.

Interns are medical school graduates who are usually not licensed to practice medicine, but are employed by hospitals to perform duties while they are gaining the additional medical education and experience required for licensure. Their duties are performed under the supervision of staff physicians of the hospital. Interns do not contract with patients to render medical treatment. As in the case of residents, interns may become the "borrowed servants" of physicians or surgeons.

The doctrine of respondeat superior also may impose liability upon a hospital for acts or omissions on the part of a nurse. Whether such liability attaches depends on whether the nurse's conduct was wrongful and whether the nurse was subject to the control of the hospital at the time the wrongful act occurred. The determination of whether the nurse's conduct was wrongful in a given situation depends on the standard of conduct to which she is expected to adhere. If at the time of the negligent conduct the nurse was subject to the control of the hospital, that nurse is an employee of the hospital and is not the "borrowed servant" of a staff physician or surgeon. Thus respondeat superior would apply.

The case of *Norton* v. *Argonaut Insurance Company,* 144 So. 2d 249 (1962), illustrates the concept of respondeat superior in the case of a nurse employed by a hospital. In this Louisiana case, a nurse questioned two physicians about a medication order she believed to be inaccurate. She did not, however, contact the patient's attending physician who had written the medication order. The nurse administered the fatal dose by injection, not realizing the order meant to specify an oral dose.

The jury found both the attending physician and the nurse negligent—the physician for writing an ambiguous medication order, the nurse for failing to question the attending physician and for administering a medication with which she was unfamiliar. The hospital did not incur liability for the physician, but did incur liability for the negligence of the nurse, a hospital employee.

The standard of care which the courts apply to the professional conduct of nurses may be contrasted with the standard of care applied to interns. In *Rush* v. *The Akron Hospital,* 82 Ohio L. Abs. 292, 171 N.E. 2d 378 (1957), the plaintiff brought an action against the hospital predicated on the alleged negligent conduct of an intern in closing wounds without thoroughly probing them and examining them, thereby leaving glass in the wounds. Plaintiff appealed the judgment, which had been rendered in favor of the defendant. On appeal it was held that the evidence was insufficient to establish negligence; therefore, the judgment for the defendant was affirmed. In articulating the standard applicable to interns the court stated:

> What is required in the case of an intern is that he should possess such skill and use such care and diligence in handling of emergency cases as capable medical college graduates serving hospitals as interns ordinarily possess under similar circumstances, having regard to the same or similar localities, and the opportunities they afford for keeping abreast with the advances in medical and surgical knowledge and science.
> *Rush* v. *Akron Hospital,* 82 Ohio L. Abs. 292, 171 N.E. 2d 378.

The court in the *Rush* case noted that it would be unreasonable to exact from an intern doing emergency work in a hospital the same high degree of skill possessed by a physician or surgeon with an extensive and constant practice in hospitals in the community. The court noted, however, that even when measured by the same standard of care applicable to a practicing physician or surgeon, the intern's conduct in this case was not negligent.

It is impossible to list all the acts and omissions that may constitute negligence on the part of a nurse and which may render a hospital liable under the doctrine of respondeat superior. Nevertheless, some examples may illustrate the circumstances under which the doctrine will apply. Cases have involved the application of overheated hot water bottles, *Norwood Hospital* v. *Brown,* 219 Ala. 445, 122 So. 411 (1929) and *Williams* v. *Pomona Valley Hospital Ass'n.*; the administration of an enema of too high a temperature, *City of Shawnee* v. *Roush,* 101 Okla. 60, 223 P. 888 (1913); the injection of incorrect medication, *Session* v. *Thomas D. Dee Memorial Hospital Ass'n.,* 94 Utah 460, 78 P. 2d 645 (1938); the failure to catheterize a patient at the intervals requested by the patient's physician, *Skidmore* v. *Oklahoma Hospital,* 137 Okla. 133, 278 P. 334 (1929); and the failure to warn a patient of danger present when lowering the patient's bed, *Welsh* v. *Mercy Hospital,* 65 Cal. App. 2d 473, 151 P. 2d 17 (1944). As we have seen in *Darling,* described earlier in this section, a hospital will also be held liable for the failure of nursing personnel to take action when it is clear that the patient's personal physician is unwilling or unable to cope with the situation that threatens the life or health of the patient.

Several courts have developed a distinction between the clerical or administrative acts a nurse performs and nursing acts involving professional skill and judgment. Under this distinction, the courts allocate liability under respondeat superior in the following way: if the act is characterized as administrative or clerical, it is the hospital's responsibility; if the act is considered medical, it becomes the surgeon's responsibility. However, the trend is away from this distinction and it is regarded as lacking a sound logical basis.

A special nurse—one hired by the patient or his agent to perform nursing services—is not generally regarded as a servant of the hospital. The hospital, therefore, is usually not held liable for the wrongful conduct of the special nurse. In some respects a special or private duty nurse might be likened to a staff physician. As with staff physicians, the hospital may require that the special nurse observe its rules as a precondition to working in the hospital. The hospital may even exclude a special nurse from practicing within the institution. The fact that the special nurse must observe hospital rules is insufficient, however, to establish a master-servant relationship between the hospital and the nurse. Under ordinary circumstances a special nurse is an employee of the patient. The hospital ordinarily has no authority to hire or fire the nurse or control the nurse's conduct on the case, but retains responsibility to protect patients from incompetent and unqualified special nurses.

Even though special nurses are employed by the patients, there are certain circumstances in which the hospital may be held liable where these nurses are negligent in the performance of administrative duties required by the hospital. Moreover, use of the designation "special nurse" does not preclude the nurse from being held an employee or agent of the hospital under certain circumstances. Where the facts of the situation indicate that a master-servant relationship exists between the hospital and the special nurse, the usual doctrine of respondeat superior may impose liability upon the hospital for the nurse's wrongful conduct. Thus in *Emory University* v. *Shadburn,* 47 Ga. App. 643, 171 S.E. 192 (1933) aff'd., 180 Ga. 595, 180 S.E. 137 (1935), the court, emphasizing that the nurse was procured and paid through the hospital, said:

> Where an application in behalf of the patient is made to the hospital to furnish to the patient a special nurse, and a special nurse is selected and procured by the hospital and placed in charge of the patient, notwithstanding the services of the nurse may be specially charged for by the hospital and paid for by the patient, but where the hospital itself is paid for the services of the nurse and the hospital afterwards settles with the nurse, the inference is authorized that the special nurse is the agent of the hospital to care for and look after the patient; and where the injuries received by the patient in jumping out of the window of the hospital under the conditions referred to are caused from any negligence of the nurse in leaving the patient alone, such negligence is imputable to the hospital.
> *Emory University* v. *Shadburn,* 171 S.E. 192 at 193.

The mere fact that a patient pays the special nurse has been held not to be conclusive evidence that the special nurse was not the employee of the hospital. Whether or not an employer-employee relationship exists, which determines the applicability of respondeat superior, is a matter to be determined by the jury under proper instructions.

A general hospital frequently contracts with physicians or a group of physicians to provide emergency medical services in its emergency room. In these circumstances the question of liability in the case of a negligence action, and whether or not respondeat superior applies, becomes crucial. In *Mduba* v. *Benedictine Hospital*, 384 N.Y.S. 2d 527 (App. Div., 1976), a New York appellate court held a hospital responsible for the negligence of a physician who operated its emergency room on a contract basis. Notwithstanding the actual contract between physician and hospital, the court said the hospital exercised enough control over the operation of its emergency room to render it liable—under the doctrine of respondeat superior—for the physician's failure to administer a blood transfusion in time to prevent a patient from going into shock. Control was found because the doctor had to conduct the operation of the emergency room in accordance with the hospital board's rules and regulations. The court also noted that the hospital guaranteed the doctor $25,000 a year and provided clerical help for billing patients. In addition, doctors' fees were based on rates set forth in the contract.

The court stated, moreover, that even if the doctor was an independent contractor it would have found the hospital responsible since the decedent entered the hospital for treatment and the hospital undertook to render that treatment. Patients entering the hospital through the emergency room could properly assume that the treating doctors and staff were acting on behalf of the hospital. The court felt that these patients should not be bound by secret limitations of a private contract between hospital and doctor—this in spite of the fact that the contract stated that the hospital was desirous of operating the emergency room on a contract and not an employee basis.

In a later case relying on *Mduba*, a New York trial court held that while a hospital is responsible for the negligent performance of doctors and staff it has hired and furnished to an injured patient, that responsibility does not absolve a negligent doctor from liability to the patient. In *Magwood* v. *Jewish Hospital and Medical Center of Brooklyn*, 408 N.Y.S. 2d 983 (Sup. Ct., 1978), the court clarified that the patient has recourse to the hospital as well as to the physician. Furthermore, lacking a clear, express agreement by the hospital to indemnify a doctor for a malpractice judgment against him, this court declared that it would imply no such indemnification obligation.

In *Hollingsworth* v. *Georgia Osteopathic Hospital*, 245 S.E. 2d 60 (Ga. App., 1978), the appellate court held that an oral contract between a hospital and a physician for provision of emergency room services created a question of fact, and thus trial should be held to determine whether the doctor was an employee or an independent contractor. The court noted that although the contract did not purport to control specific procedures the physician used in emergency room coverage, it did require regular attendance there, it did provide for a set amount of compensation per day in addition to patient fees received, and it did require the physician to perform all duties in accordance with existing professional standards.

A similar result was reached in *Mehlman* v. *Powell,* 46 U.S.L.W. 2227 (Md., Oct. 28, 1977), where the court, invoking an apparent agent theory, stressed the hospital's control over independently contracted emergency room physicians by virtue of admitting procedures (the emergency room physician did not have authority to admit patients to the hospital), billing processes (the hospital handled billing for emergency room services), and facility regulations. In addition to procedural control, the court noted that the location of the emergency room in the hospital's main building created the appearance of a master-servant relationship between hospital and physician. Therefore, in holding the hospital vicariously liable for emergency room malpractice, Maryland's highest court declared that the hospital "represented to the decedent that the staff of the [hospital] emergency room were its employees thereby causing the decedent to rely on the skill of the emergency staff, and that the hospital is consequently liable to the decedent as if the emergency room staff were its employees" *Mehlman* v. *Powell,* 46 U.S.L.W. 2227.

In a similar case, *Adamski* v. *Tacoma General Hospital,* 20 Wash. App. 98, 579 P. 2d 970 (Wash. App., 1978), a Washington appeals court also relied partially on a theory of apparent agency to allow suit against a hospital for the negligence of a physician-employee of a corporation that contracted with the hospital to provide its emergency room coverage. Without deciding whether the emergency room physician was an agent of the hospital or an independent contractor, the court noted that the doctor's services were an integral part of the hospital's operation and the doctor might, therefore, be deemed an actual agent of the hospital. Moreover, even if no actual agency were found to exist, the court stated that the unrebutted circumstances surrounding the emergency room treatment, including the doctor's use of patient instruction forms that contained the hospital's name, might support an inference that emergency room personnel were "held out" as hospital employees. This would constitute an element of the apparent agency theory. The court felt that people who avail themselves of hospital facilities expect that it is the hospital who will attempt to cure them, not that its nurses or other employees will act on their own responsibility. Thus the court decided that the case could not be decided by summary judgment, but would have to go to trial.

Basically, the "holding out" or "ostensible agent" doctrine provides that a hospital may be liable for the actions of an individual who is not an employee if the hospital has cloaked an independent contractor with indicia of apparent authority to act in behalf of the hospital.

In the Maryland case of *Thomas* v. *Corso,* 265 Md. 84, 288 A. 2d 379 (1972), the court sustained a verdict against the hospital and a physician. The patient, who had been hit by a car, was taken to the hospital emergency room. Although the patient was in shock and had low blood pressure, a physician did not personally attend to him. A nurse in the emergency department made two telephone calls to the physician who was providing on-call coverage, one call upon admission of the patient and one call just before the patient died. Nevertheless, the physician did not arrive at the hospital until just after the patient died. The court reasoned that expert testimony was not even necessary to establish what common sense indicated—that is, that a patient who had been struck by a car may have suffered internal injuries and should have been evaluated and treated by a physician. Lack of attention in such a case is not reasonable care by any standard. The concurrent negligence of the nurse who failed to contact the on-call physician after the patient's condition had worsened did not relieve the physician of his liability for failure to come to the emergency room at once. Rather, under the doctrine of respondeat superior, the nurse's negligence was a basis for holding the hospital liable as well.

To summarize, the doctrine of respondeat superior imposes liability upon the hospital for the torts of its employees which occur during the furtherance of the employer's enterprise. Imposing liability in this manner is justified because the burden of recompensing the plaintiff is borne more easily by the employer. Furthermore, in theory, the employer will be motivated to supervise employees more closely.

Another automobile accident emergency case, *Citizen's Hospital Association* v. *Schoulin,* 288 Ala. 741, 262 So. 2d 303 (1972), had a result similar to that reached in the *Thomas* case. In this case, the automobile accident victim sued the hospital and the attending physician for their negligence in failing to discover and properly treat his injuries. The court held the hospital liable through its nurse for failing to communicate all the patient's symptoms to the on-call physician, for failing to have x-rays and other diagnostic tests made as directed by the physician, and for failing to keep the patient in the hospital.

Another case on negligent staff communication and consultation is *Ramsey* v. *Physicians Memorial Hospital, Inc.* 36 Md. App. 42, 373 A. 2d 26 (1977). In this case an appellate court imposed liability on a hospital for a hospital-employed nurse's negligence by omission. Two infant brothers with symptoms of high fever and chest and head rashes were admitted for emergency room treatment. Although the mother told the nurse that she had removed ticks from one child, the nurse failed to so inform the attending physician. Subsequently one child died of Rocky Mountain Spotted Fever, which had been misdiagnosed as measles. Because the nurse's negligence was a contributing proximate cause of one child's death and of the other child's serious illness, the court concluded that the hospital was liable under the doctrine of respondeat superior. The court reasoned that the nurse's negligent omission was made within the scope of her hospital employment.

Some courts attach great importance to the terms specified in the hospital-physician contract, in order to determine whether a physician is an independent contractor or a hospital employee. This is shown in *Badeaux* v. *East Jefferson General Hospital,* 364 S. 2d 1348 (La., 1978). The facts reveal that a five-year-old child was brought to the emergency room of the defendant hospital suffering from high fever, headache, and neck and back pain. After examining the child, the emergency room physician discharged him. The child was brought back to the hospital later the same day in a coma. He was hospitalized, but died approximately one week later of meningitis. The mother of the child brought suit, alleging that the hospital was liable for the negligence of the emergency room physician because that physician was acting as the agent of the hospital. The trial court rendered judgment in favor of the hospital. An appeal was brought, but the appellate court affirmed the judgment of the lower court. It found the defendant hospital not liable because the emergency room physician was acting as an independent contractor. However, the plaintiff had not filed any sworn supported documents as he should have under the court rules.

The contract between the hospital and the group of emergency physicians was introduced into evidence by the hospital. This contract clearly delineated the responsibility of the hospital and that of the physicians. The contract contained a disclaimer stating that the emergency room group's agents and employees were not hospital agents or employees. The contract contained no provisions for hospital control or supervision over the emergency room physicians. However, the contract did require that the emergency room physicians be members of the hospital staff, and the hospital did reserve the right to designate removal of individual doctors from the emergency service.

Examining the contract together with other evidence that showed that the emergency room physicians were acting independently and not as agents or employees of the hospital, the court said:

> When the Affidavit of the Assistant Administrator and a Contract between the Hospital and the Emergency Room Corporation were considered, and in the absence of countervailing affidavits or supporting documents we conclude, that as a matter of law, no liability exists on the part of the hospital in this case for the alleged negligent acts of the assigned Emergency Room physician.

> *Badeaux* v. *East Jefferson General Hospital,* 364 S. 2d
> 1348 (La., 1978).

A result similar to that in the *Badeaux* case was reached in *Pogue* v. *Hospital Authority of DeKalb County*, 170 S.E. 2d 53 (Court of Appeals of Georgia, 1969). In this case the court carefully examined the contract between the hospital and the DeKalb Emergency Group, a partnership composed of the defendant doctor and others. Because the hospital authority had no control over the actions of the members of the partnership, the appellate court had no difficulty in affirming the judgment in favor of the hospital authority, refusing to hold the hospital liable for the alleged negligence of the defendant physician. This held in spite of the fact that the contract provided that services were to be performed to the satisfaction of the hospital, subject to surveillance by medical staff of the hospital, and in accordance with good medical practice. The contract also provided for an administrative liaison between the partnership and hospital authority. (Compare *Mduba* v. *Benedictine Hospital.*) However, the court felt that this agreement did not give the hospital the right to direct specific medical techniques employed in rendering the services. The court also noted that the agreement specifically designated the partnership as an independent contractor.

Because of the variety of ways hospitals choose to provide emergency medical coverage, there are always shades of gray between the clear case of a physician employed by the hospital (as in the case of a resident or intern) and the attending physician who is clearly an independent contractor. In each case that reaches a court, the facts will have to be analyzed carefully to determine whether respondeat superior applies to hold the hospital liable for the negligence of the emergency room physician.

Even though the contract provisions deal with the duties of the physicians by delineating which patients the physicians will treat, the standard of medical practice to be provided, and the surveillance of the treatment by the hospital medical staff, these provisions do not necessarily constitute control by the hospital sufficient to modify the independent contractor relationship set forth in the contract. Recent cases, however, indicate the courts are inclined to give less weight to the provisions of the "insulating" contracts between the hospital and contracting emergency room physicians and are inclined to hold both hospital and those physicians liable on the basis of the public's reliance on the hospital and its chosen professional personnel. Whether the hospital has exercised the requisite control over the emergency department physician is a matter that must be determined according to the facts as they are presented in each case.

As mentioned earlier in this chapter, an injured patient may sue for breach of contract rather than sue for negligence, although damages for negligence would ordinarily be higher than those for breach of contract. In some states hospitals are still immune from liability for negligence. These states are those that have chosen not to follow the lead of the Illinois *Darling* case on charitable immunity. Sometimes the patient can sue in contract for attention and treatment.

This was attempted in two separate cases, in different states, with widely disparate results. The attempt was successful in Alabama, *Berry* v. *Druid City Hospital Board,* 333 So. 2d 796 (Ala., 1976), where the state supreme court ruled that a hospital's acceptance of a patient in its emergency room could give rise to such a contract. The facts in this case reveal that the patient had "blacked out" and was taken by ambulance to the city hospital. There she was admitted to the emergency room, transferred to a treatment table, but not strapped down. Left unattended, she fainted again and apparently fell off the table, incurring injuries to her shoulder and pelvic areas. In allowing the case to proceed under a breach of implied contract theory (implied by the actions of the parties), the court rejected the rationale of earlier decisions barring contract actions when the facts also supported a negligence suit. Thus the plaintiff was able to avoid the hospital's claim of governmental immunity from malpractice suits. The court further stated that the distinctions previously made between the negligent failure to perform an agreed-upon act, and the performance of that act in a negligent manner, were artificial and unduly limiting. The court concluded that so long as the injured patient stated sufficient facts to establish the breach of a valid contract and the plaintiff's performance of that contract, the suit should be allowed to proceed.

In Kansas, however, the patient's suit was dismissed. The Supreme Court of Kansas followed the traditional rule that distinguishes suits based on tort (i.e., negligence) from those based on contract, and precluded the latter—for injuries stemming from negligent conduct—even if those injuries flowed also from a breach of contract. In dismissing the suit, *Malone* v. *University of Kansas Medical Center,* 220 Kan. 371, 552 P. 2d 885 (1976), the court noted that an injury based on negligence occurs whenever a provider of services fails to meet the duties imposed on that provider by law. In this case a pregnant woman was treated for an alleged infection on one day and was back at the hospital for a ruptured uterus the next day. Subsequently a total abdominal hysterectomy was performed without her consent. The patient's complaint that the hospital and physicians were negligent by providing incomplete, incompetent, and unauthorized treatment amounted to a claim that the medical center failed to satisfy the standard of care expected of all hospitals and physicians in the state. The remedy for such conduct lies in an action based on negligence only. The court thus followed the rule that a plaintiff cannot characterize a tort action as one in contract in order to avoid the bar of governmental immunity from tort suits. Thus no matter how incompetently the hospital acted, it was immune from suit for malpractice on either the tort or contract theory.

In *Green* v. *Hospital Building Authority of the City of Bessemer,* 294 Ala. 467, 318 So. 2d 701 (Ala., 1975), a plaintiff brought an action in contract against a hospital for breach of an implied promise to use reasonable care in furnishing services. The action arose after a hospital attendant closed a door on the plaintiff's hand. Under Alabama law, the hospital was immune from liability for negligence. The state supreme court affirmed the lower court's decision to grant summary judgment for the hospital. The court stated simply that the law would not imply a promise on the part of a hospital to use due care in attending patients in the hospital because the hospital was statutorily immune from suits. One may ask whether such immunity encourages carelessness.

Suits in contract do not pose as much threat to hospitals and emergency department staff members as do suits for negligence. Consequently, in trying to avoid liability, every attempt should be made to decrease the risk of negligence.

Statute of Limitations

The statute of limitations is addressed to the time period in which a plaintiff must bring a cause of action or forever be barred from bringing suit. It can be classified as a defense because it can be raised as such by the defendant. Statutes of limitations vary from state to state and are often specific as to the cause of action. Generally, the statute of limitations for a negligence action is two to three years. For contract actions the statute of limitations is usually six years. Some states have enacted statutes of limitations specifically for malpractice actions, and these generally are for two or three years.

The important element to grasp is when the time period actually commences. Some statutes begin running as of the date the incident occurred, whereas others are more liberal and do not begin to run until the plaintiff actually discovers or should have discovered an injury or harm.

In states having special statutes of limitations applicable to medical malpractice actions, these usually are limited to acts of negligence by physicians. Unless such statutes specifically include within their purview personal injury actions arising out of hospital care or acts of negligence by nurses, such statutes do not apply to hospitals and nurses. This is because hospitals and nurses are not licensed to practice medicine. This general principle applies except when a hospital is being sued on the basis of respondeat superior and the injury is alleged to have occurred as a result of an employee's medical malpractice.

As mentioned earlier, the statute of limitations can be raised as a defense, but in most jurisdictions a defendant must affirmatively plead the statute of limitations to avail himself or herself of its benefit. Failure to raise the statute as an affirmative defense is considered a waiver of that defense by the defendant.

Despite the fact that statutes of limitations are applicable specifically to malpractice actions and do not generally apply to actions against a hospital for personal injury, the rules that apply to medical malpractice action limitation statutes also may be applied to determine when the statute begins to run in an action against a hospital for personal injury.

The purpose of statutes of limitations is twofold: (1) it is against public policy to allow the threat of a lawsuit to last forever, and (2) it is against public policy to have the courts hear stale claims. Both reasons have merit. However, malpractice cases involve considerations that do not generally arise in other types of personal injury actions. For example, the patient may not be aware of the malpractice when it occurs; perhaps the injury may not produce an immediately noticeable effect, or perhaps the injury is a result of a foreign object being left inside a patient's body. Under such circumstances, application of the general rule that the statute of limitations begins to run when the wrongful act is committed may bar otherwise meritorious claims and leave an injured plaintiff with no legal recourse.

Thus approximately half of the jurisdictions have adopted rules to ameliorate some hardships of the general rule. Some jurisdictions have adopted the "discovery" rule, under which the statute of limitations does not commence to run until the wrongful act is discovered or, with reasonable diligence, should have been discovered. In others, the statute does not begin to run until the termination of the physician-patient relationship.

In *Pearl* v. *Lesnick,* 278 N.Y.S. 2d 237, 224 N.E. 2d 739 (1967), the plaintiff argued that she had consented only to a biopsy and not to the performed radical mastectomy. The court allowed use of the two-year assault statute of limitations for an intentional tort rather than the six-year statute for breach of contract. In Louisiana, however, a lawsuit based on an alleged failure to obtain informed consent is governed by the statute of limitations for negligence actions. In *Lombardo* v. *Argonaut Insurance Co.,* 354 So. 2d 731 (La. App., 1978), the court dismissed a patient's suit against a surgeon because the suit was not brought within a year following the operation, as required for "suits based on tort" (such as malpractice). The suit had been initiated within the longer ten-year period allowed for contract actions.

In *O'Bryant* v. *Starkman,* 53 Ill. App. 3d 991, 369 N.E. 2d 215 (1977), the plaintiff requested treatment from the defendant physician for an injured knee. The physician released the patient without having taken any x-rays and without having given any treatment. The patient later sought treatment at the emergency room of a Chicago hospital, where her condition was diagnosed as a dislocated knee. When surgery was performed to reduce the dislocation, the surgeon discovered a fractured kneecap. The plaintiff brought a suit against the defendant physician, alleging medical malpractice. However, suit was brought 19 days after the two-year statute of limitations that governed such actions in Illinois had run out. The trial court dismissed the action. The plaintiff appealed, but the appellate court affirmed the judgment of the lower court, stating: "The purpose of a statute of limitations is to encourage diligence in the initiation of actions and to discourage the assertion of stale claims. The Trial Court, therefore, correctly granted the defendant's motion to dismiss the complaint" *O'Bryant* v. *Starkman,* 369 N.E. 2d 215 at 216.

The importance of the timing of the discovery of the harm or injury is illustrated in *Bridgford* v. *U.S.,* 550 F. 2d 978 (1977). Here the U.S. Court of Appeals for the Fourth Circuit held that the two-year statute of limitations governing claims against the United States under the Federal Tort Claims Act should not preclude a suit against the government in which the claimant had no reasonable basis to believe during this two-year period that he had been negligently treated or that such treatment would later cause substantial injury. Therefore, the court held that a patient's 1972 suit for damages, allegedly caused in 1964 by the negligent performance of a vein stripping operation, was not barred by time. The court reasoned that the patient's knowledge of possible nominal damage immediately following the operation was not the same as his understanding six years later of the full extent of the damage. A claim against the government does not accrue "until a claimant had had a reasonable opportunity to discover all of the essential elements of a possible cause of action— duty, breach, causation, damages . . ." *Bridgford* v. *U.S.* 550 F. 2d 978 at 982.

The statute of limitations for malpractice may be avoided by a patient if the patient charges lack of consent to treatment. Except in emergencies, an assault and battery occurs when a patient's consent is not obtained prior to the rendering of treatment. The statute of limitations for assault is usually longer than that for malpractice. In *Karash* v. *Pigott,* 530 S.W. 2d 775 (Tenn., 1975), the plaintiffs had originally filed a malpractice complaint alleging strict liability and negligence in the administration of a blood transfusion. The Circuit Court of Shelby County denied a motion to amend the complaint to include a charge of assault and battery based on lack of consent. On appeal, the Tennessee Supreme Court held that, because both the original complaint and the proposed amendment arose out of and were part of the same conduct— namely, the transfusion—the amendment would be allowed even though the amendment itself was proposed after the one-year statute of limitations had run out.

As can be seen, an understanding of basic legal tenets helps those in the delivery of health services to understand the interface of law and patient care. The following chapter will focus on specific areas of legal concern in emergency care, beginning with the large issue of emergency and nonemergency situations.

NOTES

1. Joint Commission on Accreditation of Hospitals, *Accreditation Manual for Hospitals,* February 1978 ed. (Chicago: JCAH, 1978), p. 15.

2. Joint Commission on Accreditation of Hospitals, *Accreditation Manual for Hospitals,* 1980 ed. (Chicago: JCAH, 1979), p. 23.

3. William L. Prosser, *Handbook of the Law of Torts,* 4th ed. (St. Paul, Minn.: West Publishing Co., 1971), p. 213.

Chapter 2

Emergency versus Nonemergency Care

Over the past few decades there has been a phenomenal increase in visits to emergency departments. Hospitals have, by necessity, increased their emergency staff and their facilities to meet this demand. During the 1950s emergency room visits doubled, from approximately nine million visits in 1954 to twice that in 1958. That number doubled again ten years later. In 1968 statistics record 35,729,801 visits to emergency rooms. At this rate, by 1984 emergency room visits will approximate 160 million.[1]

There are various reasons for this marked increase in the use of emergency departments among the general public. Among the reasons are the following: (1) the decrease in the number of general practitioners of medicine, and the attendant decrease in the number of physicians willing to make house calls; (2) the availability of service provided by emergency rooms which, for the most part, are open 24 hours a day, 365 days a year; and probably most important, (3) the fact that the general public sees the emergency room as a neighborhood health center, with the cost of the visit covered by insurance.

At present the number of emergency visits is approximately twice the number of hospital admissions. Some studies show admissions to hospital beds via the emergency room as being between 30 and 50 percent. In other words, a significant number of admissions are unplanned, and this number is growing. This is because the number of actual emergency admissions to hospitals has remained relatively constant, but the number of emergency room visits has increased so dramatically that emergency room admissions are accounting for a greater proportion of total hospital admissions.

The role of the emergency room of a general hospital is changing, and this change has been evident over the past few decades. Traditionally the emergency room served to treat trauma or sudden injury. There are still many professionals who refer to the emergency room as the "accident room." The United States Public Health Service estimates that each day trauma is responsible for the death of 310 Americans, the injury of 137,000, the permanent impairment of 1,100, and the confinement of 32,000 to bed.[2] An emergency department may serve many other functions—depending on the size of the hospital, its location, and other variables—but few emergency departments fail to see their primary role as caring for the person with a sudden injury.

In addition to the traditional role, the emergency department has increasingly become an outpatient center and backup center. These roles are for the most part, but certainly not always, geared to handling nonemergency cases. Some writers have stated that because emergency departments do not share the public's view that their service includes primary care, they are not equipped to handle this nonemergency type care as well as they are equipped to handle the traumatic cases.

CURRENT TERMINOLOGY

The American Hospital Association (AHA) has published definitions on emergency care, as follows:

Emergency—An emergency is any condition that—in the opinion of the patient, his family, or whoever assumes the responsibility of bringing the patient to the hospital—requires immediate medical attention. This condition continues until a determination has been made by a health care professional that the patient's life or well-being is not threatened.

True Emergency—A true emergency is any condition clinically determined to require immediate medical care. Such conditions range from those requiring extensive immediate care and admission to the hospital to those that are diagnostic problems and may or may not require admission after work-up and observation.[3]

In addition, the American Hospital Association has published current hospital terminology for classifying patients who present themselves for care at emergency departments. These classifications include:

Emergent—Requires immediate medical attention. Delay is harmful to patient. Disorder is acute and potentially threatens life or function.

Urgent—Requires medical attention within a few hours. In danger if not attended. Disorder is acute but not necessarily severe.

Nonurgent—Does not require the resources of an emergency service. Disorder is minor or nonacute.

Scheduled Procedure—Planned in advance.[4]

The AHA recommends that hospitals count all visits made in each of these four classifications to arrive at a total for emergency patient visits.

In addition to these terms for care, AHA has defined the following:

Emergency Care System—The term emergency care system denotes a community or regional network of services that provide for detection and reporting of medical emergencies, initial care at the scene, transportation and care en route to a medical facility, and care of the patient until he is discharged, referred, or admitted for definitive medical care.

Hospital—The hospital is viewed as an organizational entity composed of a governing board, a staff (medical and nonmedical), and an administrative structure. The term hospital applies to that organizational entity.

Hospital Emergency Department—The term emergency department signifies the facilities and services provided primarily for the management of outpatients coming to the hospital for treatment of conditions clinically or considered by the patient or his representative to require immediate medical care in the hospital environment. The term is to be interpreted as synonymous with such terms as emergency room, accident room and casualty room.

Triage—Prompt, brief medical evaluation of all incoming patients to determine the nature of the problem, the level of urgency, the identification of the kind of service needed, and assignment for emergency attention.[5]

TRIAGE

Triage is a method of rapidly classifying emergency cases on the basis of the urgency of treatment that is needed. Clearly, this is an important function. There is increasing questioning as to whether triage is an exclusive function of physicians. To date there is no legal ruling that states that triage is a medical practice and therefore cannot be performed by health professionals who are not physicians. Indeed, in many emergency rooms triage is handled by emergency nurses, and there are many in the emergency health field who believe that a trained nurse can handle triage very well so long as there is adequate medical supervision and so long as the triage function is limited to seeing that patients are routed to and evaluated by physicians. In some of the emergency departments that use nurses for triage, these nurses work under standing orders from a physician.

In support of the argument that triage can be performed well by nonphysicians, especially nurses, proponents point to the screening duties of medical corpsmen in the armed forces. Indeed, this is where the concept of triage originated. Supporters also point to the fact that nurses perform triage in clinics and physicians' offices.

In determining whether triage in their emergency department has to be performed only by physicians, hospital administrators and governing boards must consider several factors: (1) the kinds of cases usually seen in the emergency department—that is, whether or not the hospital sees a large or small number of severely and critically injured persons; (2) the availability of capable personnel (both physicians and nonphysicians) trained to perform triage; (3) the legalities involved in the use of physicians or nonphysicians; and (4) the financial implications and staff employment arrangements that result from using physicians in this role. Clearly, the answer will not be the same for all hospitals. Until the professional associations (such as the American Hospital Association) issue some definitive recommendation, or a clear legal ruling is rendered, hospitals should seek to have triage performed by persons most competent and able in this area.

The performance of triage becomes more and more important with the increased use of emergency departments for both emergencies and nonemergencies. It can be argued that use of the emergency department as a source of primary care dilutes or hampers the emergency staff's ability to give optimum care to true emergencies. Clearly, there is a danger that in placing increased demand on existing staff and facilities, the standard of care may be compromised.

Nevertheless, so long as nonemergency care or primary care patients present themselves for treatment, they must be evaluated. Additionally, so long as the public is willing to use the emergency departments for primary care, these departments will continue to have a large percentage of nonemergency cases listed as emergency room visits.

Each hospital needs to look back at its own community to understand why the public has decided to use the emergency department for nonemergency care. Only then can the hospital determine how to handle this problem. A conference on hospital outpatient care, sponsored by the United States Public Health Service and held by the American Hospital Association, came up with the following recommendation:

> Hospitals are encouraged to experiment with various patterns of organizations for ambulatory services, including hospital-based physicians, group practice (prepaid or fee-for-service), interdisciplinary teams, expanded roles for existing personnel, and development of new types of personnel.[6]

One might hazard a guess that the public will choose any competent care at the lowest out-of-pocket expense to the patient.

Conference participants acknowledged that we need to develop better methods to handle individuals who present themselves at emergency departments for nonemergency conditions. One suggestion was to have a common entrance for both the true emergency and the nonemergency patients. A rapid triage system would direct patients to a separate area set up for each of the two classifications—two areas with separate staffing.

Presently, the handling of nonemergency patients varies a great deal. Some hospitals have outpatient and drop-in clinics to which they can refer patients. If these clinics are operated 24 hours a day, it is relatively easy to refer patients immediately. However, more often these clinics do not have such wide service hours, so patients must be referred and asked to return when the clinic is open.

Another method of disposition of nonemergency patients is to refer them to private physicians. This is not always easy to do. Many persons come to emergency departments because they cannot reach their own physician or because their own private physician has sent them to the emergency department. With a 50 percent decrease in the number of physicians in private practice over the past several decades, this will continue to be a problem.

A third method of disposition is to treat fully all persons requesting treatment. This, of course, puts a tremendous strain on the staff and the facility and leads to the problem of overutilization of the department and a probable lowered standard of care.

One final method of disposition seems to hold more promise. This is to evaluate the patient and make an appointment for a more thorough evaluation and treatment at an off-peak time in the department.

If hospitals truly want to limit the use of their emergency departments to patients with true emergencies, they must try to restructure the hospital to meet the public need for primary care. This could be done in a variety of ways. One way would be to develop ambulatory care facilities within the hospital setting. In order to significantly reduce the use of the emergency room, these ambulatory care facilities would have to be staffed and equipped to provide comprehensive service at convenient times and locations. Preferably, they would be open on weekends, holidays, and during evening hours. In addition, hospitals should look into the possibility of developing community and neighborhood health centers, health vans, and outpost ambulatory units operated by the hospitals themselves.

It is important for hospitals to determine how to define the emergency department. Some studies on the use of emergency departments reveal that approximately 80 percent of emergency room visits are not true emergencies at all. Some estimate that true emergencies account for only five percent of emergency room visits.[7]

In 1972 in one detailed study of the use of an emergency department of a general hospital in upstate New York, it was found that 49 percent of emergency department visits were for abrasions, contusions, cuts, or minor or major burns. Additionally, only in ten percent of the visits were patients admitted to the hospital. The author concluded that "true emergency is relatively infrequent in this study. Emergencies of a minor nature occur in relatively large numbers."[8]

More recent studies have shown a much greater number of hospital admissions from the emergency department. A detailed study of a Northeastern hospital in 1978 found that "While total hospital admissions over the nine-year period have leveled off, the trend of emergency department admissions continues to increase steadily. While such admissions accounted for only 20.4 percent of total hospital admissions in 1966, this figure is more than 50 percent in 1974 at this institution."[9]

Thus it is incumbent on each hospital's governing board to look at the patterns of utilization in the emergency department to determine how service can be improved, expanded, contracted, or generally altered to meet community needs.

One commentator has strongly suggested that hospitals develop ambulatory care. William C. Van Lopik, Fellow: Hospital Financial Management Association, makes a direct correlation between the decrease in private medical practice visits (from nearly 100 percent to 50 percent in the last century) and the increase in hospital ambulatory care visits. Van Lopik states, "From 1967 through 1970 hospital outpatient service increased 22 percent compared to 8 percent for inpatients. Most of this growth was in emergency and, especially, ancillary services. Clinic services decreased proportionately. Emergency rooms have ceased to provide emergency services. They have evolved into medical clinics."[10] Van Lopik concludes by stating:

> Sociological and technological changes require organized delivery of ambulatory care, which hospitals have been increasingly providing. Hospitals face difficult problems in expanding their roles beyond emergency room and indigent clinic services. But they have great capacities and unique capabilities to be the best providers of quality ambulatory care at the lowest possible cost if allowed to do so.

Applications of marketing, production and financial skills in addition to medical skills are needed to successfully overcome barriers to deliver ambulatory care.[11]

RESPONSIBILITY OF EMERGENCY DEPARTMENTS TO SEE ALL PATIENTS WHO PRESENT THEMSELVES FOR TREATMENT

The rapid increase in the number of people who present themselves to emergency departments for treatment—including those who do not have true emergency situations—raises the problem of the hospital's responsibility to treat any and all who appear and seek care. The traditional rule, in law, has been that hospitals are not required to admit everyone who seeks admission. Regardless of this traditional rule, hospitals may not legally refuse to admit patients on a discriminatory basis. In emergency situations, a different rule applies: where an emergency exists, a hospital with an emergency department is required to provide service.

The problem is that at present there is no clear definition of an emergency. Generally speaking, an emergency is an illness or injury that could result in death or permanent bodily impairment. Examples of emergency conditions requiring the immediate attention of a physician to prevent loss of life include the following:

- massive hemorrhage from major vessels (heavy bleeding)

- cardiac arrest (heart attack)

- cessation or acute embarrassment of respiration (breathing stopped)

- profound shock from any cause (collapse with increased heart rate and white skin tone)

- rapidly acting poison

- anaphylactic reactions (allergic response)

- acute epidural hemorrhage (collection of blood within brain following head injury)

- acute overwhelming bacteremia and toxemia (release of bacteria into bloodstream; decrease in blood pressure; increase in temperature)

- severe head injuries

- penetrating wound of the pleura or pericardium (heart or lung wound)

- rupture of an abdominal viscus (any internal organ of abdomen)

- acute psychotic states (sudden and complete change in personality).[12]

In some states—including California, Florida, Illinois, New York, Tennessee, and Wyoming—statutes have been enacted requiring certain private hospitals to render emergency care to persons seeking it. California Ch. 1219, S.B. No. 888 (Laws 1977), requires each county exceeding a population of 100,000 to provide emergency medical personnel to county hospitals or to hospitals contracting with the county to provide emergency services. These persons, who are to be present or on call at all times, are also to be trained in examining sexual assault victims.

All the states that have enacted such legislation impose penalties for noncompliance. The more typical penalty is a fine. However, the New York law threatens to suspend or revoke the hospital's license. The Florida statute provides for imprisoning violators for up to 60 days.

The oldest such statute was enacted in Illinois in 1927, and it has been a forerunner for statutory action in other states. The Illinois statute requires that every licensed hospital providing general medical and surgical services in the state shall provide a hospital emergency service and must furnish such hospital emergency service to any applicant who suffers from an injury or acute medical condition that is liable to cause death or severe injury or serious illness. Clearly, this statute was aimed at emergency care and is not really addressed to the large number of nonurgent cases presently seen in emergency rooms.

In the majority of states, there is no statutory duty on hospitals to render emergency care. Thus in these states the common law must be consulted when courts are faced with questions of the hospital's duty to provide emergency care. The major case dealing with this question is *Wilmington General Hospital* v. *Manlove,* 54 Del. 15, 174 A. 2d 135 (1961). Here the emergency department nurse refused to admit a seriously ill four-month-old child who was suffering from diarrhea and an elevated temperature. The nurse refused because the child was already under the care of a private physician and the parents did not have authorization from that physician. The nurse claimed that hospital policy required she first contact the private physician before administering treatment, because there was a danger that the hospital's medication might conflict with that of the attending physician. Although the nurse tried to contact the infant's doctor, she was unable to do so. The parents took the child home, where he died that afternoon.

The Delaware Supreme Court ruled that the hospital might be liable for refusal to treat the infant. The basis of the court's decision was the patient's reliance on the hospital's custom to render aid to persons with "unmistakable emergencies." The rationale is that in seeking aid and having it refused, the individual is worse off for having treatment delayed. Thus the court affirmed the denial of a summary judgment and sent the case back for further proceedings to determine whether the hospital was negligent in not responding to a true emergency.

The reliance theory advanced in *Manlove* has been followed by courts in other states. In essence courts are finding that hospitals that hold themselves out to the community as providers of emergency care and treatment have assumed a duty to provide that care and treatment to all individuals who present themselves and request aid. In cases following the rule of *Manlove,* courts have emphasized the reliance theory and have repudiated the traditional rule that hospitals are free to choose patients they will treat *when an emergency exists.*[13, 14]

For hospitals struggling to determine their legal obligations, there remains the problem of defining an emergency. The courts have not shown consistency on this issue. In states with statutory definitions of emergency, the courts will use those definitions. However, in the majority of states where no such definition exists, the courts must look at the specifics of the case being litigated to determine whether an emergency existed.

Thus while it is well established that hospitals are not under a legal duty to treat individuals who present themselves for nonemergency, ambulatory care, hospitals are duty-bound to evaluate all individuals to determine whether or not emergency care is indicated. The evaluation should be based on whether refusing treatment aggravates the individual's condition, thereby posing a threat to life or well-being.

> The operation and maintenance of the hospital emergency department clearly creates one of the highest liability exposures of any activity within a hospital. To the extent to which facilities are available, it is much more prudent to err on the side of caution and to retain or admit questionable patients than to have the actions of hospital personnel judged after the fact to determine the adequacy of the emergency diagnosis and screening.[15]

There are two other issues involved in determining the responsibility of emergency departments to see all patients who present themselves for treatment: (1) hospital policies to contact an individual's private physician before rendering treatment, and (2) conditioning treatment on an individual's ability to pay.

Some hospitals have unwritten policies that prohibit emergency room physicians from treating patients who seek care if those patients are patients of physicians on the hospital's admitting staff, unless the private physician is contacted and gives permission. This restriction is not good practice and hospitals should avoid it. Emergency department policies and procedures should state clearly that it is the responsibility of the emergency room physician to give needed treatment. Unwritten policies that deviate from written policies would have no force.

On the issue of conditioning emergency care on one's ability to pay, it seems apparent from case law that this is not allowed. Although hospitals have been upheld in requiring payment for routing admissions, the same rule does not apply in emergency situations. In *Mercy Medical Center of Oshkosh* v. *Winnebago County,* 58 Wis. 321, 206 N.W. 2d 198 (1973), the Wisconsin Supreme Court stated:

> It would shock the public conscience if a person in need of medical emergency aid would be turned down at the door of a hospital having emergency service because that person could not at that moment assure payment for the service.
> *Mercy Medical Center of Oshkosh* v. *Winnebago County,* 58 Wis. 321, 206 N.W. 2d 198 at 201.

EMERGENCY DEPARTMENT EXPOSURE TO LIABILITY

The emergency department is at risk in terms of exposure to legal liability. Principally this is because of the kinds of injuries and illnesses seen and treated, the urgency with which decisions on treatment often must be made, and the availability of staff and facilities to handle the demand for service.

Interestingly, a 1971 Maryland study on malpractice revealed that emergency departments were not high risk areas in a hospital, and that indeed more malpractice emerged from physicians' private offices and in-hospital departments than from emergency departments.[16]

Nevertheless, the constant pressure and tension in a busy emergency room does not allow much time for reflection on a diagnosis, evaluation, or consultation on the method of treatment. Thus it always is imperative that the emergency department be adequately staffed by highly skilled personnel who can provide the best possible care.

There are ways to increase the efficiency of emergency departments and thereby reduce their exposure to liability. Obviously, a first step is to provide enough of the best available staff. Another aid is to draft policies and procedures that clearly delineate the function of the emergency department. Some commentators have written that frequently emergency departments try to do too much. If the demand on the emergency department is so great that the staff cannot handle that demand adequately and efficiently, rules prohibiting certain nonemergency functions should be enacted. One rule could prohibit the use of the emergency room by private physicians for treatment of their private patients. Another rule could prohibit its use for minor elective surgical procedures and for elective psychiatric work. In fact, elective procedures of any kind should be discouraged or scheduled only for off-peak times. This would effectively curtail overuse of the department. If this policy was coupled with the establishment of outpatient clinics for the large number of persons seeking nonemergency care, the traffic, tension, and confusion would be reduced significantly, thereby permitting the staff to concentrate on true emergencies.

The use of an emergency department ombudsman has helped some hospitals facilitate the operation of the emergency room. In one study on the impact of such an ombudsman, the authors concluded:

> The ... study indicates that an ombudsman can alleviate some of the chronic complaints that plague emergency departments: long waiting, the perceived impersonality of harried staff members, and a lack of information and emotional support. Although length of visit was not significantly reduced, patients and their companions were less concerned about waiting time and were better able to understand and accept delays. The presence of the ombudsman decreased the proportion of respondents who approached staff members with a question or a request, thereby freeing staff to concentrate on treatment. The ombudsman was enthusiastically received by patients, who described positive experience of emotional support and increased information. The ombudsman's activity also eliminated below average or poor ratings of medical care and overall services in the emergency department. Contact with the ombudsman was associated with increased understanding of instructions and more frequent follow-up.
>
> The study results indicate that the services of an ombudsman are a useful adjunct to technical skills in the delivery of emergency care and that use of an ombudsman can be a preventive measure against common complaints. The large volume of visits to community hospital emergency departments, in numbers that far exceed annual admissions, suggests that an ombudsman has a potential impact on improving the image of these institutions within the community.[17]

ABANDONMENT

As discussed earlier, no individual who reports to an emergency department should be refused treatment. Simply by presenting oneself to an emergency department, an individual signifies a request for care. To prevent legal liability for abandonment (failure to take necessary steps for follow-up care, when such

t should be a policy of every emergency department to ....-up instructions to patients. This could take the form of a simple ....uction sheet or follow-up letter to the patient. Whether a letter or form is sent, a copy of that letter or form should be made a permanent part of the patient's record.

The form or letter should clearly signify that the care given was on an emergency basis and that further medical care is needed. It would be helpful to detail the possible results of lack of follow-up care. See Exhibit 2-1 for an example of such a form.

The legal theory of abandonment is grounded on the fact that no physician is compelled legally to accept any request for service. However, once a physician-patient relationship is established by advice, examination, treatment, or counseling, the physician is responsible for the continued care of the patient until that responsibility is assumed by another physician. It is unethical and legally dangerous for a physician to establish a physician-patient relationship and then refuse to continue treatment. If the patient truly needs medical care, and the physician who has established a physician-patient relationship refuses to continue care or treatment, that physician is liable for a civil action based on abandonment.

Although abandonment is an action against a physician rather than against a hospital, the hospital could be held liable under the doctrine of respondeat superior if the physician is an employee of the hospital. Additionally, if the physician is not a hospital employee but an independent contractor, the holding-out doctrine might be used to hold a hospital liable if the physician has

---

Exhibit 2-1 Sample Form for Follow-Up Care

INSTRUCTIONS FOR FOLLOW-UP CARE

The examination and care you have been rendered was on an emergency basis only and cannot replace or substitute for total medical care. For your protection, it is recommended that you follow the instruction outlined below to prevent any complications.

☐ Report at once to your private physician.
☐ Report at once to_____Clinic.
☐ Contact your private physician or clinic for an appointment on_____ _____.
☐Report back to this Emergency Department on_____.

Date_____   Signed_____, M.D.

been given apparent authority by the hospital to act on its behalf, since in this case it would appear to the public that the physician was employed by the hospital. Thus it is essential that once treatment is initiated, it not be discontinued so long as the patient needs continuing care.

GOOD SAMARITAN LEGISLATION

In 1959 California became the first state to enact legislation protecting "Good Samaritans" from liability while rendering aid in emergency situations. Since then, every state (including the District of Columbia and the Virgin Islands) has enacted its own version of this law. Only Puerto Rico does not have a Good Samaritan law.

For emergency department staff the important point to remember is that the Good Samaritan acts do not apply to them. This is because the basic purpose of this legislation is to encourage trained persons to render emergency assistance to victims of accidents or other emergencies by protecting these persons from suit or, at least, from liability.

More than half of the states require that the emergency aid provided must be rendered gratuitously. Generally, this means without compensation. The relatively few court decisions in this area have held that the statute does not provide protection for in-hospital aid or in cases where the individual had a duty to render aid. Duty would be implied in cases where emergency department personnel were employed for compensation.

In addition to the requirement that the aid be rendered gratuitously, some state laws specifically define Good Samaritan acts as those performed outside of the "normal course of employment." Thus, on-duty time is not included in actions protected by Good Samaritan statutes. Additionally, some of the state laws specifically exclude coverage when aid is rendered in hospitals, and some state laws define "at the scene" as excluding hospitals, a doctor's office, or a place with medical equipment.

From these exclusions it is easy to see the intent of the legislatures that enacted these laws. Legislators were concerned about emergency care at the scene of an accident, especially a highway accident.

Whether or not these laws are necessary and whether or not they actually encourage emergency assistance is a matter of great controversy among commentators and legal writers. The controversy is not aided by the fact that much of the statutory language is ambiguous and needs clarification.

Very few court decisions have dealt with Good Samaritan acts, but two recent cases did involve these laws. In *Guerrero* v. *Copper Queen Hospital,* 112 Ariz. 104, 537 P. 2d 1329 (1975), the court held that the Good Samaritan Act did not apply because the care provided was rendered in a hospital. A more recent case, *Colby* v. *Schwartz,* 78 Cal. App. 3d 885, 144 Cal. Rptr. 624 (1978), dealt specifically with emergency department staff members. This case involved a malpractice action against emergency room physicians. The California Court of Appeals rejected the contention of the defendant physicians that the California Good Samaritan Statute applied to a hospital emergency room, thereby rendering them immune to suit for negligence. In fact, the court held that the Good Samaritan Act did not apply because the care was provided in a hospital. The court refused to extend the statute to physicians "practicing within their area of expertise and with all of the benefits of full hospital facilities," and held that it was not the intent of the law to protect in-hospital emergency room physicians.

The fact that *Colby* was a case involving physicians limits its holding to physicians only. However, one can predict that a similar ruling will be made in a future court case involving nurses or other emergency room health personnel. Thus it is imperative that emergency room personnel recognize that Good Samaritan acts do not apply to their on-duty practice.

ISSUES OF CONSENT

Issues of consent will be dealt with comprehensively in Chapter 4. However, we want to touch on this topic here since a large number of visits to emergency departments are nonemergency in nature, and a true emergency can change the general legal rule concerning consent.

The general rule on consent is that every patient has a legal right to be treated only with his or her consent. There is an exception to this rule in the case of an emergency. In an emergency medical care can be given without consent to save a life or prevent permanent bodily injury. Thus if it is impossible to obtain consent and delaying treatment would jeopardize life, it is legally correct to render treatment without consent. When the emergency department staff is dealing with a nonurgent case, consent is essential.

One of the problems currently facing emergency departments is the use of blanket consent forms. These forms are legally ineffective when they authorize department staff to do anything necessary or anything deemed advisable. Courts have viewed these blanket forms as worthless when they do not include designation of the problem and the specific treatment authorized by the patient.

When a decision is made that an emergency exists and consent cannot be obtained, the decision to proceed with treatment should be made by a physician and that decision should be documented. Documentation can be in the manner of a form (such as Exhibit 2-2).

Exhibit 2-2 Sample Form Indicating Decision to Proceed with Treatment

Date _____ Time _____

We, the undersigned physicians, licensed to practice in the State of_____, do hereby certify that in our opinion_____
(patient
_____, _____, is in need of immediate treatment to preserve
  name)   (age)
life and/or to prevent permanent bodily injury or deformity.

We further certify that repeated unsuccessful attempts have been made for a reasonable time to contact the parents, spouse, or legal guardian of the patient named above, and that further delay in rendering treatment will, in our judgment, seriously increase the danger to the patient's life, health, and well-being.

_____Witness   _____,M.D.
_____Witness   _____,M.D.

There are certain kinds of cases that often appear in emergency departments for which there are legal risks regardless of what steps the staff members take. For example, consider the case of a drunken patient who comes to the emergency department in obvious need of care but refuses to be examined or give consent to any treatment. A case of this sort presents a conflict in rules. On the one hand, the patient has presented herself or himself for treatment. Obviously she or he must want treatment or she or he would not have appeared. Sometimes, the situation is further complicated because the patient has been brought in by friends and has not come in of his or her own accord. On the other hand, this same patient may have a severe laceration that requires suturing to prevent excessive bleeding.

The strict legal answer would dictate that treatment cannot be given without the patient's consent. To delay treatment until a court-appointed guardian can give consent is not much help to emergency department staff. Of course, if the person were unconscious, consent would be implied by the law. But the person we are discussing is conscious, though inebriated. Thus rendering treatment without consent raises the risk of a lawsuit for assault and battery.

In this kind of situation, the emergency room physician must balance the risks: treatment risks suit for battery, and nontreatment risks suit for failure to treat (which could result in death or disability). On balance, it would be preferable to render treatment even though there is a clear legal risk. It is helpful in such a case to have documentation by more than one physician that treatment is needed.

Inability to Comprehend English

In some emergency departments, especially those in general hospitals located in large cities with sizable immigrant populations, the department is heavily used by people for whom English is not the primary language. Without a doubt, people cannot possibly give informed consent if they cannot comprehend what is being explained to them. To date, the courts have not held physicians liable for failure to obtain informed consent when the failure resulted from the patient's inability to speak or comprehend English. This is not to say that a future case would not find liability. Thus, although currently there is no court ruling or statute that requires informed consent be explained and obtained in a patient's native language, it is good practice to make provisions for non-English-speaking patients. In emergency departments where many visits are made by people of the same ethnic group, it makes sense to have forms and instructions in that language. An interpreter on staff would also be helpful.

What happens when the staff member does not speak English as a primary language? In some emergency departments, interns and residents regularly rotate through the department. When these staff members have difficulty with the English language, there are innumerable communication problems—not only with patients but with other staff members. This problem is, of course, compounded when patients also do not communicate well in English. One of the authors saw this problem firsthand with an intern from the Philippines and a patient from Puerto Rico. If such a communication problem exists or is likely to arise, policies should be drafted to eliminate or minimize the problem.

Statutory Consent

A battery is committed if a sample of a person's breath, blood, urine, or other bodily substance is taken without consent, even if the person is brought to the emergency department by the police on suspicion of drunken driving. Both the hospital and the staff member who draws the sample may be liable for an unauthorized touching.

In some states the motor vehicle laws provide that the acceptance of the privilege of driving on the highways implies a person's consent to furnish a sample of blood or urine for chemical analysis if that person is charged with driving while intoxicated. Generally where statutes imply authorization of a test for intoxication, an assault and battery action will not be upheld. It is not clear, however, whether an action for battery would apply if the test were conducted after the driver voiced objections. The Kansas statute, for example, assumes consent if a person accepts the privilege of driving, but it specifically acknowledges that such consent may be withdrawn and that the person may refuse to submit to the test. Several other states make the same provision.

Some states have also dealt with the issue of implied consent in cases where the person is unconscious at the time a sample of blood, urine, or breath is taken. One state has specifically provided that an unconscious person is considered not to have withdrawn consent to any such test. Another state has provided that, at least for the purposes of a criminal or civil case, it would be conclusively presumed that the person has refused to consent to and has in fact objected to such tests. In states that have not specifically dealt with the issue of the unconscious person, the situation is not clear.

There are no reported decisions regarding the extent of hospital or personnel liability for obtaining a testing sample from a person who did not give consent when the sample was requested by a law enforcement officer. Some states have enacted statutes that imply that court action may be brought against not only the individual who obtains such a sample but also the hospital that employs that person. Other statutes protect physicians, hospitals, and hospital employees from any liability for obtaining a blood sample from a nonconsenting individual when that sample is requested by a police officer. Such a statute has been enacted in Louisiana. It provides:

> C. No person who administers any such test upon the request of a law enforcement officer as herein defined, no hospital in or with which such person is employed or otherwise associated or in which such test is administered, and no other person, firm or corporation by whom or which such person is employed or is in any way associated, shall be in any wise criminally liable for the administration of such test, or civilly liable in damages to the person tested.
> Added by Acts 1968, No. 273, § 14. Amended by
> Acts 1972, No. 534, § 1.

Such statutory protection would probably extend to physicians, hospitals, and their employees for performing a test in accordance with proper medical standards, but would not protect them from liability for negligent performance of a test resulting in injury or damages. In the absence of this statutory protection, such a procedure would constitute a battery. However, recovery would probably be limited to nominal damages unless physical harm resulted from negligent performance.

It must be recognized that even though the admission of test results as evidence against a defendant in a criminal proceeding may not violate constitutional rights, the hospital employee who draws the sample may still be liable for an unauthorized touching. There is little doubt that taking a sample of breath, blood, urine, or other bodily substance from a person brought to the hospital by the police or from a patient upon request of the police, without the consent of that person, is a technical battery. In *Bednarik* v. *Bednarik,* 18 N. J. Misc. 633, 16 A. 2d 80, 90 (1940), the court said:

> To subject a person against his will to a blood test is an assault and battery, and clearly an invasion of his personal privacy. It involves the sticking of a surgical needle into his body. Perhaps the operation is harmless in the great majority of cases, although the risk of infection is always present. But if we admit such an encroachment upon the personal immunity of an individual where in principle can we stop? . . .

If the purpose of withdrawal of a blood sample is misrepresented, consent for the procedure may not be effective, thereby making the results of the test inadmissible as evidence and establishing a basis for tort liability. In *Graves* v. *Beto,* 424 F. 2d 524, cert. denied, 400 U.S. 960 (1970), consent was given by a criminal suspect in response to a request by the police for the sample to determine intoxication. However, the authorities were actually interested in learning the suspect's blood type as part of their investigation of an alleged rape. The court said the test results were inadmissible as evidence and pointed out that the time required to obtain a proper search warrant to test for blood type would not have jeopardized the investigation because blood type, as distinguished from the alcoholic content of the blood, is a continuing condition that is not altered by the passage of time.

For its own protection a hospital is wise to ask that the patient sign a consent form such as Exhibit 2-3.

CONTRACEPTIVES

Some emergency departments are visited by patients experiencing difficulty with contraceptives. Many contraceptive clinics that operate on an outpatient basis have arrangements with emergency departments of nearby hospitals to treat their patients for complications or during hours that the clinic is closed.

The doctrine of informed consent has been administratively expanded by the Food and Drug Administration (FDA) to require that physicians who prescribe an intrauterine device (IUD) warn patients of the device's risks (42 F.R. 23772, May 10, 1977). The regulations, effective as of November 7, 1977, provide that prior to insertion of an IUD, patients be given a copy of the IUD brochure supplied by the manufacturer and have an opportunity to discuss fully with appropriate health care personnel any questions they may have regarding use of an IUD.

Exhibit 2-3 Patient Form Authorizing Blood Sample

CONSENT TO TEST

The undersigned hereby consents to the taking from him/her of a blood sample to be used for police purposes. The undersigned specifically authorizes the _____ Hospital, its agents and employees, to cooperate, permit, and assist in the taking of the blood sample, and agrees that the hospital, its agents and employees, will incur no liability whatsoever arising out of the taking of the blood sample.

Date _____   _____

Witness_____   (signature)

The patient brochure is to be divided into two sections and written in lay language. It should acquaint a patient with all information relevant to an informed decision. In the first section, covering preinsertion information, the following topics should be addressed:

- what the patient should know about the IUD

- use-effectiveness

- what the patient should tell her doctor

- adverse reactions.

In the second section, covering postinsertion information, the following topics should be discussed:

- a description of the device

- directions for its use

- a listing of side effects

- a listing of warnings

- a special warning about pregnancy with an IUD in place.

Before inserting an IUD, physicians are also required by the FDA to inform patients of contraceptive alternatives and their risks and benefits. Although the regulations do not mandate a specific formal informed consent procedure (except in the case of investigational drug IUDs), they do advise physicians to offer patients the same type of consent information as would be given in any other comparable medical procedure. In addition to the patient information requirements, the regulations set forth medical procedures that physicians should follow in selecting candidates for IUD use and recommend follow-up procedures.

The Food and Drug Administration has issued stricter labeling requirements aimed at promoting the "safe and effective" use of oral contraceptives (43 F.R. 4214, January 31, 1978). The requirements, which became effective April 3, 1978, are comparable to FDA regulations that require that informational brochures be given to IUD users. The FDA has mandated that patients receive from their pharmacist or other dispenser informational leaflets written in lay language informing users of the risks of oral contraceptives, their side effects, proper usage, effectiveness, and contraindications (i.e., conditions making their use inadvisable). The regulations also require that hospitals supply the informational leaflet to patients before administering the first oral contraceptive and every 30 days thereafter, as long as therapy continues.

Similarly, the widespread medical use of drug products containing estrogen has prompted the FDA to require disclosure to patients of the risks inherent in utilizing these products (42 F.R. 37641, July 22, 1977). The FDA now requires that each prescription-dispensed estrogen product be accompanied by a label containing the following information: the drug's name and its manufacturer's name and address, a general statement regarding the drug's proper usage, a warning of its known risks, a discussion of the drug's possible adverse side effects and danger signs, and a reminder to the user that the product is prescribed solely for the user's own medical treatment and must not be given to others.

The label, to be supplied by the drug manufacturer, should be given to the patient at the time the prescription is dispensed. Hospitals will be acting in compliance with this regulation by furnishing a label to each patient prior to receipt of the first dose and at 30-day intervals thereafter, so long as estrogen thereapy continues.

CHILD ABUSE

Child abuse will be dealt with more fully in Chapter 8. It will, however, be mentioned in this chapter as it is frequently seen in emergency departments. Victims of child abuse should be treated, even though child abuse does not always technically fit the definition of a true emergency.

Child abuse cases can be detected by emergency department staff in a variety of ways. Some methods of detection are covered in an excellent article by the head nurse of a Spokane, Washington hospital emergency department.

For example, child abuse may be suspected when the parents show loss of control or fear of losing control, overreact or underreact to the seriousness of the child's injury, show unrealistic expectations of the child, are reluctant to give a medical or case history, give a history that does not explain the child's injury, give a contradictory history, or use several hospitals for the child's treatment.

Child abuse may be suspected when the child shows an unexplained injury; overall poor health or poor care; an unusually fearful appearance; dehydration or malnourishment without obvious cause; or evidence of having received inappropriate food, drink, or drugs.[18]

SEXUAL ASSAULT

Victims of sexual assault, including rape, are frequently seen in the emergency departments of general hospitals. Although their cases do not usually fit the definition of a true emergency as that term is strictly defined, it is essential that these patients be treated skillfully, as every one represents a potential court case. (There are, of course, times when sexual assault involves minors, making it an element of child abuse.)

Until very recently, the legal definition of rape excluded acts by a husband against his wife. Traditionally, in legal terms, rape has been defined as the unlawful carnal knowledge of a woman by a man, forcibly and against her will. However, the Model Penal Code definition reflects typical state laws more accurately:

Section 213.1 Rape and Related Offenses.

(1)   Rape. A male who has sexual intercourse with a female not his wife is guilty of rape if:
   (a)   he compels her to submit by force or by threat of imminent death, serious bodily injury, extreme pain or kidnapping, to be inflicted by anyone; or
   (b)   he has substantially impaired her power to appraise or control her conduct by administering or employing without her knowledge drugs, intoxicants or other means for the purpose of preventing resistance; or
   (c)   the female is unconscious; or
   (d)   the female is less than 10 years old.

Rape is a felony of the second degree unless (i) in the course thereof the actor inflicts serious bodily injury upon anyone, or (ii) the victim was not a voluntary social companion of the actor upon the occasion of the crime and had not previously permitted him sexual liberties, in which cases the offense is a felony of the first degree. Sexual intercourse includes intercourse per os or per anum, with some penetration however slight; emission is not required.

(2)   Gross Sexual Imposition. A male who has sexual intercourse with a female not his wife commits a felony of the third degree if:
    (a)   he compels her to submit by any threat that would prevent resistance by a woman of ordinary resolution; or
    (b)   he knows that she suffers from a mental disease or defect which renders her incapable of appraising the nature of her conduct; or
    (c)   he knows that she is unaware that a sexual act is being committed upon her or that she submits because she falsely supposes that he is her husband.

In the past few years, as a result of the prodding of feminists, legislators have begun to take a hard look at the restrictive definitions of rape. Consequently they have begun to acknowledge that state laws do not include men as rape victims, although there is no doubt that men are victims of rape. There has also been increasing recognition that rape does occur between married people. For example, suppose a couple has been separated for a number of years but has never obtained a divorce. If the husband assaults and rapes the wife, he could not be charged and prosecuted for rape as they are still legally married.

Because some states have recently broadened the legal definitions of rape and sexual assault, it is important for emergency room staff members to familiarize themselves with the local laws and regulations that cover these crimes. Emergency department personnel should also know what is meant by the following:

Statutory Rape—coitus with a female below the age of consent—commonly, but not always, 16 years of age. Typically, the female has consented, but the laws deem her too young to be able to consent.

Sexual Molestation—noncoital sexual contact without consent.

Deviate Sexual Intercourse—Commonly, this term refers to anal or oral sex between members of the same or opposite sex and also includes sex between a human male or female and a beast. The present trend is to make all private deviate sexual acts between consenting adults noncriminal acts.

The requirements for reporting sexual assaults to the police vary from state to state. However, if a patient alleges rape and consents to it being reported, the police should be notified immediately. If the hospital staff suspects rape, but the patient does not allege it, an "authorization for release of information" should be filled out. If the patient is a minor—that is, under the age of 18—it is likely there will be a duty to report the assault to the appropriate state officials, under the child abuse or battered child laws.

Because every alleged sexual assault represents a potential court case, the emergency room staff should recognize that the patient's medical record will probably be subpoenaed. Therefore, it is important to have the necessary consent forms for treatment (including collection of specimens and estrogen therapy, if indicated), photographs, and release of information ready to give to the proper authorities. In addition, it is important to document the patient's history carefully and completely. The history should include the date and time of the alleged act, any injuries, and the patient's emotional state.

Physical examination should be performed as soon as possible. Record the general appearance of the patient, including bruises, ripped clothing, evidence of bleeding, and any signs of trauma. If there is injury to any bodily part other than the genitals, this should be noted. Venereal disease testing should be done. A pregnancy test should be performed if there is a possibility of pregnancy. The cervix and vagina should be inspected with a nonlubricated (but water-moistened) speculum. Vaginal aspiration should be performed by inserting 10cc of normal saline into the vagina and withdrawing a sample with a vaginal pipette. There should also be an immediate examination for the presence of sperm. With the high percentage of men who have undergone vasectomy, sperm may not be found. In any case, tests for seminal fluid should be performed. The specimens collected should be labeled accurately and carefully and should be sent to the laboratory. The specimens must not be lost, destroyed, or mismanaged in any way as they will be needed as evidence by the prosecuting attorney should suit be brought.

Clothing, photographs, and other forms of evidence should be given to the police, who should give the patient a receipt detailing the items. The receipt should be included in the hospital record, and a notation should be made in the record of the transfer of the items.

Patients should be followed to determine if pregnancy or venereal disease occurs. Emergency room staff should offer referrals for psychological counseling. Patients should be encouraged to return to the emergency department for additional treatment, if necessary.

NOTES

1. W. C. Van Lopik, "Ambulatory Care: Fertile Field for Hospital Growth," *Hospital Financial Management* 32, no. 8 (August 1978), p. 27.

2. *Hospital Law Manual* (Germantown, Md.: November 1977).

3. American Hospital Association, *Emergency Services—The Hospital Emergency Department in an Emergency Care System* (Chicago: AHA, 1972), p. vi.

4. Ibid., pp. vi and viii.

5. Ibid., p. viii.

6. American Hospital Association, *Outpatient Health Care—The Role of Hospitals* (Chicago: AHA, 1969).

7. William R. Kucera, "Narrow Definition of 'Emergency' Can Spell 'Litigation'," *Hospital Medical Staff* 7, no. 9 (September 1978), p. 21.

8. Arthur R. Jacobs et al., "Emergency Room Crisis and Challenge," *New York State Journal of Medicine* (December 1972).

9. Samuel B. Webb, Jr., et al., "Emergency Department and Inpatient Service: A Symbiotic Relationship?" *Journal of Ambulatory Care Management,* no. 2 (April 1978), p. 81.

10. William C. Van Lopik, "Ambulatory Care: Fertile Field for Hospital Growth," p. 26.

11. Ibid., p. 28.

12. Thomas Flint et al., *Emergency Treatment and Management,* 5th ed. (Philadelphia, London, Toronto: W. B. Saunder Co., 1975), p. 690.

13. Powers, "Hospital Emergency Service and the Open Door," *Michigan Law Review* 66 (1968), p. 1455.

14. William R. Kucera, "Narrow Definition of 'Emergency' Can Spell 'Litigation'," pp. 21-27.

15. Ibid., p. 27.

16. James E. George, "Medicolegal Problems of Emergency Medicine," in *Principles and Practice of Emergency Medicine,* Vol. II (George Schwartz et al. (eds.), (Philadelphia, London, Toronto: W. B. Saunders Co., 1978), p. 1495.

17. Dorothy S. Lane and David Evans, "Study Measures Impact of Emergency Department Ombudsman," *Hospitals* 52 (February 1978), p. 99.

18. Tenna Cael, "Child Abuse: Hospital Team and Public Agencies Help Patients and Parents," *Hospitals* 52, no. 22 (November 1978), p. 135.

Part II

Admissions and Transfers

Admission Policies and Problems

This chapter deals with admission policies—both in the hospital in general, and specifically in the emergency room. We will discuss the problems that result from the lack of clear, comprehensive, up-to-date policies on admission of patients for treatment. We will look at what happens when perfectly adequate policies are not communicated. Additionally, we will discuss the use of triage and its attendant responsibilities.

Generally, there are no legal problems in admitting a patient to a general hospital when that patient's attending physician (who has admitting privileges with the hospital) has made prior arrangements. However, there may be problems when a hospital does not want to admit a person for treatment and finds itself in the difficult position of turning away a person who has come seeking aid.

The courts have hesitated to veer from the traditional view that no individual has a positive right to be admitted to a hospital. This traditional rule has application to all three types of hospitals: charitable, government, and proprietary. Although courts have tended to adhere to this traditional view, they have found other reasons to impose a duty on hospitals to admit persons for care and treatment under various circumstances.

Discrimination in admission of patients or segregation of patients on racial grounds is illegal for any hospital that receives financial assistance from the federal government. A government hospital cannot legally discriminate on the basis of race because its operation is state action and therefore would be in violation of the Fourteenth Amendment to the Constitution. Nongovernment hospitals can also be subject to the provisions of the Fourteenth Amendment if they are involved in state activities.

In addition to the prohibitions of the Fourteenth Amendment, the Department of Health and Human Services (HHS) has guidelines that require that no racial discrimination be practiced by any hospital receiving money under

ε λ

orted by HHS. This would include all hospitals receiving
ider Medicare, Title 18 of the Social Security Act.

about every hospital in the United States is prohibited from
ial segregation in its admission policies.

GOVERNMENT HOSPITALS

Government hospitals are by definition creatures of some unit of government, and their chief concern is service to the population of the jurisdiction within that unit. Thus whether a person is entitled to admission to a particular government hospital is contingent on the statute that established that hospital.

The statutes, in some cases but not all, establish government hospitals for the benefit of the indigent sick residents of the area. Indigency is usually defined as the inability of the individual, or those persons who are legally responsible for the individual's support, to pay for hospital care. In such a hospital admission procedures necessarily address the applicant's financial status to determine eligibility for admission.

Those government hospitals that are not limited by statute to the care of the medically indigent are legally authorized to admit both paying and nonpaying patients. Admission would still be contingent on the patient meeting the legal requirements of admission—and, of course, the patient's physical condition must necessitate hospital care. Government hospitals that operate as general hospitals may legally limit their facilities, as do nongovernment hospitals, by including or excluding persons on the basis of the medical problem. Thus it is common for government hospitals to limit their care and treatment procedures to specified categories of illness, such as mental illness or tuberculosis. Some statutes provide that where there is need to render hospital care to either preserve life or prevent permanent bodily harm, the hospital may dispense with complying with the statutory requirements for admission. Once a government hospital has begun to render care to an individual seeking emergency assistance, it must continue treatment in accordance with the applicable standard of care.

Clearly then, although government hospitals can refuse to treat those applicants who do not meet the statutory definition of those who have a right to treatment, they do have a duty to extend reasonable care to persons who present themselves for assistance and are in need of immediate attention. In these cases, government hospitals must abide by the same rules that govern nongovernment hospitals.

NONGOVERNMENT HOSPITALS

Under common law, a person has no right to aid and assistance from another person or from a hospital. The law has never imposed a duty on an uninvolved stranger to come to the aid of another person, even if that person was in obvious need of help. In *La Juene Road Hospital, Inc.* v. *Watson,* 171 So. 2d 202, 203 (Dist. Ct. of App. of Fla., 1965), the court stated "Harsh as this rule may sound, it is permissible for a private hospital to reject for whatever reason, or no reason at all, any applicant for medical and hospital services."

However, the law has carved several judicial exceptions to this rule. Once control over a person is exercised, simply stating that no duty to act existed does not relieve an individual or a hospital of liability if the person is harmed as the result of unreasonable conduct. By exercising control, a hospital does become subject to the duty of reasonable care. Much of the litigation over when this duty to act arises has involved charitable rather than government or proprietary hospitals, but there is no reason to believe that noncharitable hospitals would be judged differently.

The second exception to the traditional rule involves the conduct of a person who, although not necessarily negligent, is responsible for an injury. Once an injury occurs, there is a legal duty to either make a reasonable attempt to give aid and assistance or to desist from aggravating the original injury. If the original injury is aggravated, liability will be imposed for the aggravation only, and not for both the original and the aggravated injury.

A charitable or private hospital, as opposed to a government hospital created by statute, is under no duty or obligation to give care or treatment to any particular person. However, there are times when a hospital may be duty-bound to give assistance and care to persons presenting themselves for aid, even though these individuals have not been admitted through formal admitting procedures. For example, if a patient or visitor became ill or injured on the premises of a hospital, it would be the hospital's duty to render competent aid and assistance.

EMERGENCY SITUATIONS

The original Hill-Burton legislation mandated that each state submit a plan providing for adequate hospitals and other facilities to serve persons residing within its boundaries. In 1970 the act was amended to include provisions for emergency service. Each hospital's emergency department would be considered part of the state plan to provide emergency care for its citizens. As a result there is an increasing amount of state legislation that imposes on hospitals a duty to provide emeregency services. Some of these statutes implicitly or explicitly require that hospitals provide some degree of emergency services. However, the courts have not yet clearly mandated that any person seeking emergency services must be admitted by the hospital at which that person presents himself or herself.

As a case in point, in *Hill* v. *Ohio County,* 468 S.W. 2d 306 (1971), a pregnant woman approached a nurse working at her desk in the Ohio County Hospital in Kentucky. The woman stated she did not believe she could get back to her physician in Illinois before she delivered her baby. The nurse called two of the four members of the hospital's medical staff to authorize admission but both refused to do so. That night, after the expectant mother left the hospital, she delivered her baby at home, unattended. She was taken by ambulance to Owensboro Hospital, about 25 miles from Ohio County Hospital, but she was dead on arrival. The court held that both the hospital and the nurse were entitled to dismissal of the suit as a matter of law. The court held:

> In the instant case, the decedent was not admitted to the hospital nor was the element of critical emergency apparent. The hospital nurse acted in accordance with valid rules for admission to the facility. The uncontradicted facts demonstrate that no breach of duty by the hospital occurred. . . .
>
> *Hill* v. *Ohio County,* 468 S.W. 2d 306, 309 (1971).

A Delaware case, *Wilmington General Hospital* v. *Manlove,* 54 Del. 15, 174 A. 2d 135 (1961), concerned the liability of a private hospital for the death of an infant who was refused treatment at the hospital's emergency ward. The Delaware Supreme Court held that where a private hospital maintains an emergency unit, a refusal to render service to a person in an "unmistakable emergency" may give rise to liability when such refusal causes injury.

The facts in *Manlove* reveal that on January 4, 1959, Darien E. Manlove, the deceased infant, then four months old, developed diarrhea. The next morning his parents consulted their doctor. That evening the baby's temperature was above normal. They called the physician again, and the doctor prescribed an antibiotic which he had delivered by a pharmacy. The morning of January 6th, the child's mother took the baby to the physician's office. The physician prescribed a liquid diet and some medication. The next morning, the baby's temperature was 102 degrees. The parents, knowing that Wednesday was the doctor's day off, and determined to seek additional medical assistance, took their infant to the emergency ward of the Wilmington General Hospital.

At the hospital, the parents told the nurse on duty at the reception desk of the emergency ward that the child had not slept for two nights, had a continuously high temperature, and had diarrhea. The father explained that the child was under the care of a physician and showed her the medication prescribed. The nurse explained to the parents that the hospital could not give treatment because the child was under the care of a physician, and there would be danger that the hospital's medication might conflict with that of the attending physician. The nurse did not examine the child, take his temperature, feel his forehead, or look down his throat. The child was not in convulsions and was not coughing or crying. There was no discernible area of body tenderness.

The nurse tried unsuccessfully to get in touch with the attending physician. She suggested that the parents bring the baby to the pediatric clinic the next morning, Thursday.

The parents took the baby home. The mother reached the attending physician by phone and made an appointment for eight o'clock that evening. At eight minutes past three o'clock that afternoon, the baby died of bronchial pneumonia.

Suit was brought against the hospital for wrongful death. The complaint charged negligence in failing to render emergency assistance, in failing to examine the baby, in refusing to advise the intern about the child or permit the parents to consult the intern, and in failing to follow reasonable and humane hospital procedure for the treatment of emergency cases. The defendant hospital denied negligence and contended that, pursuant to its established rules and community practice, plaintiff was advised by its employee that it was unable to accept the infant for care.

There were two issues here: (1) whether the hospital was under any duty to furnish medical treatment to any applicant for it, even in an emergency; and (2) whether the existence of an apparent emergency was a material fact in dispute.

The court pointed out that since the defendant institution was privately owned and operated, it would follow logically that its trustees or governing board alone had the right to determine who should be admitted as patients. The court also stated that no other rule would be sensible or workable. It cited authority for this rule, but then questioned the applicability of the rule to patients applying for treatment at an emergency ward.

The court dismissed the defendant hospital's claim that it followed a rule or practice to refuse medical aid to persons already under the care of a physician, because the rule seemed to be a general rule of admission; it was not a specific rule for emergency cases. Moreover, the court felt that it implicitly recognized that in case of unmistakable emergency there was some duty on the part of the hospital to help.

The court then turned to the important question of whether the hospital had any duty to give treatment in an emergency case—i.e., one obviously demanding immediate attention. The court stressed that a private hospital is under no legal obligation to the public to maintain an emergency ward. However, the

court questioned whether a hospital that did maintain an emergency room—
with the community thus relying on that custom—should have the right,
without any reason, to refuse treatment to an applicant who had relied on that
custom. The court noted that refusing to render treatment might well result
in worsening the condition of the injured person because of the time lost in
a useless attempt to obtain medical aid.

The court then considered the duty of the nurse to one applying for admission as an emergency case. Obviously, the court stated, if an emergency is
claimed, someone on behalf of the hospital must make a *prima facie* decision
on whether it exists. The question of what constitutes an "unmistakable emergency" itself raises a difficult issue of fact. Thus the state supreme court sent
the case back for further proceedings to determine whether the hospital was
negligent in not determining a true emergency.

The distinction between *Manlove* and previous similar cases is the recognition by the court that a hospital, even a charitable hospital, that maintains an
emergency service may not refuse without a valid reason to give treatment to
one who appears to and, in fact, does require emergency attention. The theory
underlying this position is that because of the time lost in a useless attempt
to obtain aid at the hospital, the person's condition may deteriorate. Thus the
court applied the principle that the hospital's operation of an emergency
service constituted an invitation to those in need of aid.

In *Stanturf* v. *Sipes,* 447 S.W. 2d 558 (1969), the Missouri Supreme Court
reversed a summary judgment in favor of the defendant, a hospital administrator who had refused to allow a patient to be admitted to the hospital because
of an inability to pay a $25 admission charge, even though the money was later
offered to the hospital by a relative. The patient had suffered frostbite of both
feet. The court held that the evidence sustained findings that the hospital "was
the only hospital in the immediate area, it maintained an emergency service
and . . . plaintiff applied for emergency treatment and was refused." Furthermore, the court stated that

> the members of the public . . . had reason to rely on the hospital's
> practice, and in this case it could be found that plaintiff's condition
> was caused to be worsened by the delay resulting from the futile
> efforts, to obtain treatment from the . . . (h)ospital.
> *Stanturf* v. *Sipes,* 447 S.W. 2d 558, 562 (1969).

Another expression of the principle that all persons, even nonresidents, have
a legal right to rely on the availability of emergency services even from private
hospitals is found in *Guerrero* v. *Copper Queen Hospital,* 112 Ariz. 104, 537
P. 2d 1329 (1975). In this case suit was brought against the defendant private
hospital on behalf of two infants who were burned in their home in a border

town in Mexico and were taken to the emergency room of an Arizona hospital. The hospital refused to treat them. The plaintiff alleged that the delay caused by the refusal resulted in additional injury and prolonged the infants' convalescence. The plaintiff also alleged that the hospital had for years maintained an emergency room, that the room was for the benefit of any individual requiring emergency care, that it had been the practice of the hospital to care for any member of the public who was seriously injured, that the general public understood that any person seriously injured would receive care there, and finally, that the hospital held itself out as willing to treat any seriously injured person at the emergency room.

The trial court had sustained the hospital's demurrer, holding that the appellants had stated no cause of action. The Court of Appeals reversed, deciding that the appellants had stated a cause of action, and the Arizona Supreme Court upheld that decision. The courts rejected the traditional common law doctrine that a private hospital was not duty-bound to accept any patient. The Arizona Court of Appeals stated:

> The allegations are sufficient to state a claim for, if proven, liability on the part of a private hospital may be predicated on the refusal of service to a patient in case of an unmistakable emergency, if the patient has relied upon a well-established custom of the hospital to render aid in such a case.
>
> *Guerrero* v. *Copper Queen Hospital,* 22 Ariz. App. 611, 529 P. 2d
> 1205, 1206 (1974).

The Court of Appeals also relied on the policy of the Joint Commission on Accreditation of Hospitals when it stated:

> We should also point out that if a hospital has been accredited by the Joint Commission on Hospital Accreditation, such commission requires that its accredited hospital with emergency room facilities render emergency [care] to *all* who need it. It is *arguable* that by asking for and receiving accreditation, the hospital has undertaken a duty to the public, modifying the common law.

The Arizona Supreme Court declined to base its decision on this reasoning, although it easily could have done so. The Supreme Court upheld the decision of the Appeals Court based on its reading of the Arizona statutes and regulations. The court held that it appeared clear from these statutes and regulations that the state's public policy required a general hospital to maintain facilities to provide emergency care. Thus such a hospital in Arizona could not deny emergency care to any patient without cause.

The traditional common law rule, alluded to by the court in *Guerrero,* goes back to a 1934 Alabama case, *Birmingham Baptist Hospital* v. *Crews,* 229 Ala. 398, 157 So. 224 (1934). In *Crews* a child suffering from diphtheria was brought to a charitable hospital. The house physician rendered treatment, which consisted of swabbing the child's throat and giving her injections of antitoxin. Then the child's father was informed that the hospital did not accept patients with contagious diseases. The child was returned home by auto and died soon after.

In the suit the parents contended that the death of the child was accelerated by the weakening effect of the antitoxin, coupled with the exertion of the trip home. It was urged that, after having commenced emergency treatment, the hospital was obliged to render ordinary hospital services and should not have told the child's father to take her away.

The hospital was not held liable because the court said no duty existed to accept the patient:

> Defendant is a private corporation, and not a public institution, and owes the public no duty to accept any patient not desired by it. In this respect it is not similar to a public utility. It is not necessary to assign any reason for its refusal to accept the person for hospital service.

After pointing out that the hospital's rules prohibited the admission of contagious disease patients, the opinion further stated:

> We think that such treatment (the emergency care rendered) does not justify an inference that defendant undertook to render ordinary hospital service in violation of its rules, and so as to endanger the life or health of other patients.

> To uphold plaintiff's contention, we assume that, if defendant did not propose to render hospital service, it should have sent the child away in the desperate condition without emergency treatment, when such treatment was available and provided the only hope of recovery. The willingness of defendant to provide such treatment should not be used to its prejudice for not violating its rules and endangering other patients.
>
> *Birmingham Baptist Hospital* v. *Crews,* 159 So. 224, 225.

The foregoing case illustrates the traditional view that a person does not have a positive right to be admitted to a hospital. However, it also recognizes the distinction between the traditional view and the principle that the exercise of control might give rise to a duty on the part of the hospital to meet the appropriate standard of care. The court is reluctant, on the facts of this case, to require the hospital admit everyone, under all circumstances, in need of hospital care merely because emergency assistance is rendered. Such a requirement might conceivably inhibit hospitals from furnishing any emergency care because they fear liability.

The courts initially view a hospital and a prospective patient in much the same manner they view two ordinary persons. Thus the preceding principles may be formulated as a rule that provides that an individual has no absolute right to aid from another individual or a hospital. However, once assistance is initiated, neither an individual nor a hospital can defend unreasonable conduct on the grounds that there was no duty to act. Instead, the duty can only be discharged by conduct in accord with the appropriate standard of care.

These cases, coupled with similar trends in state legislation, indicate that hospitals would be prudent to (1)   maintain an open-door policy in emergency rooms, and (2)   furnish adequate diagnostic and treatment services for emergencies in order to avoid claims of improper rejection, transfer, or recognition of emergency cases.

REASONABLE CARE UNDER THE CIRCUMSTANCES

In deciding whether there is a duty on the part of the hospital and whether that duty has been fulfilled, a court must consider each of the following: (1)   the existence of a duty, which may arise by virtue of the hospital's exercise of control over the person, by legislative enactment, or by recognition of an invitation to the public; (2)   the nature of the services available at the hospital which would affect the hospital's ability to furnish attention; and (3)   a determination of whether the hospital had acted reasonably.

All three of these factors were discussed in *O'Neill* v. *Montefiore Hospital,* 11 App. Div. 132, 202 N.Y.S. 2d 436 (1960). A man, fearing he had suffered a heart attack, presented himself at the emergency room of a charitable hospital. His wife described his condition to the nurse in charge and requested that a physician examine him. When Mr. O'Neill mentioned his membership in the Health Insurance Plan of Greater New York (H.I.P.), the nurse noted that the hospital did not treat H.I.P. patients. A physician associated with H.I.P. was called. Mr. O'Neill spoke with the physician on the telephone, and that physician told him to go home and return when H.I.P. was open. The wife again asked the nurse to have her husband examined by a physician, but the nurse disregarded the request and told Mr. O'Neill that his family physician would see him at eight o'clock. Mr. O'Neill replied that he could be dead by eight o'clock. He returned home. While disrobing he fell to the floor and died before medical attention could be obtained.

Suit was brought against the hospital and against the H.I.P. physician. With respect to the issue of the hospital's liability, the court held that there were several fact issues that should have been presented to the jury for resolution. First, was the nurse's action in calling the physician a personal favor or had she acted as an employee of the hospital? Second, if her action did constitute an exercise of control, had she met the applicable standard of care? Third, did the nurse's refusal of the request for an examination after the telephone conversation constitute negligence? The court said:

> In this case the plaintiff's proof was prima facie sufficient to permit, but not to mandate the inference that the nurse in charge of the emergency ward undertook to provide medical attention for the deceased. In sum, this was a question of fact for the jury. It was error, therefore, to dismiss the case against the hospital at the close of the plaintiff's case.
>
> *O'Neill* v. *Montefiore Hospital,* 202 N.Y.S. 2d 436, 440.

The applicable standard of care can be ascertained by considering specific cases in which the hospitals have been held liable. Such cases have involved the failure to render reasonable patient care where examination has revealed a critical condition. For example, in a New York case, *Barcia* v. *Society of New York Hospital,* 39 Misc. 2d 526, 241 N.Y.S. 2d 373 (1963), an action was brought against the hospital for wrongful death of the decedent. Maria Barcia at the time of her death was a little over two years of age. Despite the fact that she was brought to the hospital with high blood pressure and respiratory distress, among other symptoms, she was denied hospitalization before the results of certain diagnostic tests were available. To the court this constituted a basis for finding the hospital negligent.

At the request of Dr. Valente, Maria's family physician, she was brought by her parents to the defendant hospital on May 5, 1958. They presented a note from Dr. Valente requesting that Maria be admitted and hospitalized. The admitting physician, Dr. Baum, examined Maria and over his own signature made the following entry in the hospital records: "found the following symptomology: a temperature of approximately 104.2 degrees Fahrenheit, pulse rate of 120, respiration 48 per minute, tonsils one to two times enlarged and mildly inflamed, throat red, had running nose, respiratory distress, coarse sounds in chest, rales along the border of the spine." He went on to say he found the child "looking acutely ill to a mild degree."

A throat culture was taken, along with a chest x-ray and a blood count. An examination of the wet x-ray indicated a pneumonitis in the right lower lobe of the lung posteriorly. The blood count showed the white corpuscles 20,000 or above, indicating the presence of an infection. As for the throat culture, all the experts who testified seemed to agree that the results of the throat culture could not be known for 24 hours, or, if it was hurried, in 13 hours at the very least. The parents testified that upon receipt of the blood count and wet x-ray, Dr. Baum told them Maria was not ill enough to be hospitalized and recommended that she return home. He gave a list of certain things to be done for her and drugs to be administered; he also told the parents to return her to the care of the local family doctor, Dr. Valente. All of this was noted in Dr. Baum's handwriting in the medical record.

Pursuant to the doctor's instructions, the parents took the child home. Her condition grew progressively worse, and again they called in the family doctor. He ordered her to be taken back to the defendant hospital. This time, the following morning, Maria was admitted. From the evidence, the court stated it believed every effort was made to save her life. Despite these efforts, she expired of staphylococcus aureus pneumonia.

The parents further testified that the surgeon who attended Maria, and who had the sad duty of informing them of her death, asked them why they had not brought her in sooner as he might have been able to save her. The court noted the tragic truth: that she had been brought in sooner and turned away. This poses the question of defendant's negligence. Only one of the doctors who saw the decedent testified, the family physician who had recommended her hospitalization. Dr. Baum did not testify. It was explained to the court that Dr. Baum was now believed to be in the State of Washington, beyond the jurisdiction of the court. No reason was given for failing to take his deposition. The other medical testimony was by experts. One expert, for the plaintiff, said Maria should have been taken in when presented and that it was professional negligence not to do so. The other expert for the defendant—the present head of the pediatric department of the defendant hospital—stated, not having seen the child, but from the record, he would have made the same determination as Dr. Baum. This doctor further stated that the hospital cannot accept everyone who applies for admission.

Simple addition shows two doctors who said Maria should have been hospitalized, and two who said the contrary. However, only one of these four testifiers saw the actual condition of the child at the time she was sent to the hospital, and he was the one who recommended hospitalization. Dr. Baum was not in court to defend his judgment.

In answer to the court's question, both experts conceded that in the absence of the throat culture, staphylococcus aureus pneumonia could not be ruled out. Dr. Baum did not wait for the report before sending the child away. Defendant's expert's only plea was that it would not have made any difference if the report had been known.

The court pointed out that it was not bound to accept that opinion as a matter of law and in fact rejected it. The court also noted that the defendant's expert made a valiant attempt to explain away the apparent contradiction in Dr. Baum's statement that the child was "looking acutely ill to a mild degree." The expert stated that Dr. Baum must have meant that she looked ill, but that her symptoms came on suddenly.

The court pointed out that Dr. Baum, as the duly authorized admitting physician of the defendant hospital, had the opportunity to examine and appraise the child's illness. The court also pointed out that there was sufficient proof upon which to base a finding of negligence on his part, and noted that an appropriate inference could be drawn from the failure to produce Dr. Baum at the trial or to have taken his deposition. The court then held the defendant hospital responsible for Dr. Baum's acts.

In another example, the Maryland case of *Thomas* v. *Corso,* 265 Md. 84, 288 A. 2d 379 (1972), the court sustained a verdict against the hospital and a physician. The patient, who had been hit by a car, was taken to the hospital emergency room. But a physician did not personally attend to the patient although the patient was in shock and had low blood pressure. There was some telephone contact between the nurse in the emergency department and the physician who was providing on-call coverage, but Corso was not seen by a physician until three hours after admittance, at which time the physician pronounced him dead. The court reasoned that expert testimony was not necessary to establish what common sense indicated—that a patient who had been stuck by a car might have suffered internal injuries and should have been evaluated and treated by a physician. Lack of attention in such a case is not reasonable care by any standard. The concurrent negligence of the nurse, who failed to recontact the on-call physician after the patient's condition worsened, did not relieve the physician of his liability for failure to come to the emergency room at once. Rather, under the doctrine of respondeat superior, this was a basis for holding the hospital liable as well.

In both the *Barcia* case and the *Corso* case, the courts did rely on the doctrine of respondeat superior. Once again, the doctrine of respondeat superior imposes liability upon the hospital for the torts of its employees which occur during the furtherance of the employer's enterprise. Imposing liability in this manner is justified because the burden of recompensing the injured person is borne more easily by the employer and, in theory, the employer is thus motivated to supervise employees closely.

In *Reeves* v. *North Broward Hospital District,* 91 So. 2d 307 (Fla. Dist. Ct., 1966), the plaintiff appealed from a final judgment entered in favor of the defendant. Plaintiff had brought this action for wrongful death to recover damages for the loss of support of her adult son, Eddie Lee Davis, who was taken by a fellow employee to Provident Hospital. Plaintiff's son was suffering from head pains and had to be assisted into the hospital.

The resident physician, an employee of the hospital, examined the patient and diagnosed his condition as hypertension. The doctor did not take a written medical history but did run a urine test and took the patient's blood pressure. The physician prescribed sedatives and gave some to the patient. Plaintiff's witness described the patient as being incoherent and speaking with difficulty. The examining physician was relieved by another physician who did not see or treat the patient but signed his discharge slip. That afternoon, on the return trip to the hospital, the patient died of a subdural hematoma.

The court pointed out that whether the hospital had a duty to admit Mr. Davis and render medical attention became a question of fact in view of the testimony of an expert witness, a neurosurgeon unaffiliated with the hospital, who testified that there were sufficient symptoms evident to alert a medical practitioner that a serious problem existed. The court noted that this evidence, together with the circumstances of plaintiff's leaving the hospital, was sufficient for a jury to find that the hospital employees did not exercise a reasonable standard of care. Judgment was reversed and the case was remanded for a new trial.

The applicable standard of care can also be ascertained by considering specific cases in which hospitals have not been held liable. In *Fabian* v. *Matzko*, 344 A. 2d 569, 236 Pa. S. 267 (1975), a hospital and physician moved for summary judgment in a suit against them for failing to render emergency treatment and for failing to admit a patient. The facts showed that a husband and wife contacted their family physician when the wife developed sudden intense pain and nausea. The family physician diagnosed her condition as a viral infection. Since the prescribed medication had no noticeable effect, the husband telephoned the hospital and was connected with a staff physician. The husband expressed a desire to have his wife admitted. The staff physician told him that hospital policy required that arrangements for admission be made by the family physician. The husband was unsuccessful in trying to locate the family physician in order to secure admission, and later he could not recontact the hospital staff physician.

The wife's condition seemed to improve, but two weeks later she had another attack and was admitted to the hospital. It was later discovered that the wife had sustained a cerebral hemorrhage with permanent brain damage, loss of speech, partial paralysis, loss of hearing, loss of vision, and expressive and receptive aphasia.

The husband and wife based their contention for recovery on Restatement of Torts §323, which states that if the hospital, through its staff physician, either gratuitously, or for a consideration, renders a service, it is subject to liability for the resulting physical harm from the physician's failure to exercise reasonable care in that relationship. The court rejected this contention because there was no finding that a physician-patient relationship had ever existed. Even under the broadest interpretation possible, there were no medical services offered. The staff physician only reiterated by telephone what constituted hospital policy.

The husband and wife also based their suit on the developing case law under *Wilmington General Hospital* v. *Manlove,* cited previously in this chapter. In that case, it was held that a hospital with an emergency facility has a duty to admit patients in need of care, where the patients relied upon a well established custom of the hospital to render such aid. The court in *Fabian* rejected this contention because there was no apparent emergency situation here. The staff physician had no reason to believe that the family physician's diagnosis was incorrect, that the condition was more serious than a viral infection. Neither did the husband and wife rely on any public policy toward emergency care. Had they felt the situation was truly an emergency, they would have come to the hospital. Since the couple failed to introduce sufficient evidence on their behalf, the lower court's motion for summary judgment for the defendant hospital and doctor was affirmed.

In a related case, *Campbell* v. *Mincey,* 413 F. Supp. 16 (D. Miss., 1975), a federal court in Mississippi found that a woman's normal labor did not constitute a medical emergency, and in the absence of such an emergency, the hospital staff was justified in denying her admission based on a preestablished policy that required local physician referral except in true emergency situations. Plaintiff, a black indigent, did not have a local physician who could refer, and the hospital had no physicians on call for such exigencies. She had no time to reach another hospital and was therefore forced to deliver her child in the front seat of an automobile in the hospital parking lot. The only assistance the hospital offered was to provide a sheet in which to wrap the newborn and to summon an ambulance to take mother and child to the hospital where she had received prenatal care, and where she originally was scheduled to deliver. The mother had an uncomplicated delivery, and her baby was not injured.

Plaintiff contended that this admission policy violated the hospital's statutory duty to provide care pursuant to state law and the equal protection guarantees of the United States Constitution. Although the hospital was a government hospital, the court rejected both arguments. It found, except for Mississippi Code, 1972, §41-9-17, some of the state's provisions to be merely general licensure statutes. However, under this statute there was a duty to provide care but the duty must have been established by regulations written to implement the law. The record made no mention of the existence or nonexistence of such regulations, and the federal court could not take judicial notice of or consider them.

With respect to the equal protection argument, the court reaffirmed previous holdings that the equal protection clause does not prohibit all discrimination between persons or groups of persons; that clause only precludes irrational discrimination. Furthermore, the duties in Mississippi Code, 1972, §41-9-17, were imposed upon the hospital, not upon its employees, and the hospital was not named as a party defendant in the case. The court found further that because there was no proof that the hospital's policy of treating emergency patients differently from nonemergency patients caused actual injury to patients, it must accept the considered judgment of the medical specialists and uphold hospital policy.

The court then found no evidence to support plaintiff's contention that the hospital had discriminated against her on account of race; she had been admitted for treatment during a previous pregnancy, and the hospital regularly treated more blacks than whites in its emergency room. The court also found plaintiff's indigency unrelated to the denial of care since her Medicaid card guaranteed payment of hospital bills incurred. The suit was dismissed.

Thus if it appears to a judge or jury that it should have been recognized that an emergency existed, a hospital or a physician may well be held liable for not admitting a patient.

Another case, illustrating the standard set by the Louisiana courts, is *Joyner* v. *Alton Ochsner Medical Foundation,* 230 S. 2d 913 (App. Ct., La., 1970). Here plaintiff had instituted suit for damages following treatment in the emergency room of defendant hospital for injuries sustained in an automobile accident. After trial on the merits, there was judgment in favor of all remaining defendants. Plaintiff's suit against them was dismissed. Plaintiff appealed.

On appeal, plaintiff contended there was liability on the part of the defendants because the Foundation and the Clinic (1) failed to give him proper emergency treatment and had allowed him to suffer unattended while he was in the emergency room for approximately four hours awaiting admittance to the hospital; (2) refused to admit him to the hospital for purely financial reasons after leading him to believe he would be admitted; and (3) failed to advise him that he would not be admitted to the hospital and should seek medical assistance elsewhere.

The facts revealed that following the automobile accident, plaintiff was brought to the defendant hospital's emergency room by ambulance solely because that hospital was the one closest to the scene of the accident. While plaintiff was in the emergency room the staff was extremely busy taking care of approximately 14 emergency cases that arrived during that time, as well as several other patients who had arrived previously.

Plaintiff's injuries consisted of multiple, deep facial lacerations; a possible head injury; traumatic damage to the teeth; and multiple bruises and contusions of the body, resulting in considerable loss of blood. On admission he was put on a stretcher, and a bandage of some kind was placed over his face. His blood pressure and pulse were taken and found to be in the upper normal limits. He was sent to the x-ray room where 14 different views were taken of his face, neck, and other parts of his body.

Thereafter his blood pressure and pulse were taken periodically. The blood pressure dropped progressively and Ringer's solution was given intravenously. Additional blood pressure and pulse readings were recorded. About three hours after admission, an analgesic was given along with tetanus toxoid to prevent infection. About four hours after admission to the emergency room, plaintiff was transferred to the Veteran's Administration Hospital where his injuries were treated.

Plaintiff's wife testified that, in her opinion, her husband was allowed to lie on the stretcher without proper attention and without being given medication for relief from pain. She further testified that she had had some discussions with an attendant and one of the doctors in the emergency room regarding admitting plaintiff into the defendant hospital, and she was asked for a $100 deposit for that purpose. She also testified that it was at her request that her husband was transferred to the VA hospital.

The medical testimony established that it was medically unwise to administer any form of pain-relieving medication until plaintiff's pressure had stabilized at a safe level and until the x-rays had revealed an absence of serious head injury.

The court found no merit in plaintiff's first contention that he was not given proper emergency treatment, as the record satisfied the court that proper emergency treatment had been rendered. The court then noted that plaintiff's contention that he was in the emergency room awaiting admittance to the hospital was factually incorrect. The court pointed out that plaintiff was taken to the emergency room for emergency treatment and not for the purpose of being admitted to the hospital.

The court then stated that there was no merit in plaintiff's second contention —that he was refused admittance to the defendant hospital for purely financial reasons after being led to believe that he would be admitted. The record revealed that, in accordance with the defendant hospital's policy and practice, if plaintiff's condition had been such as to require immediate admission to and treatment in the hospital he would have been admitted and treated. But, the court noted, his condition did not require such admission as an emergency measure. The court also noted that the requirement of a deposit before admission is the usual procedure among private hospitals in the area where, as here, the patient has nothing to offer for the purpose of assuring payment of hospital bills. In the court's opinion, in cases where there is no immediate need for emergency treatment, the requirement of a deposit prior to hospital admission is neither unreasonable nor improper.

The court stated that it could not understand the plaintiff's third contention —that the hospital had failed to advise him immediately upon his arrival at the emergency room that he would not be admitted to that hospital and that he should seek medical assistance elsewhere. The court noted that the plaintiff was brought to the emergency room for emergency treatment and not for the purpose of being admitted to the hospital. It was therefore unreasonable to complain that upon arrival he was given needed emergency treatment and not told to go elsewhere. Judgment of the lower court was affirmed.

It should be noted that in *Joyner* as well as in other cases the court gave great weight to the policies and practices of hospitals. Thus it is imperative that hospitals have clearly written policies to govern admission of patients in general and admission of patients to emergency departments in particular.

The importance of adherence to departmental policies is an essential protection against malpractice suits. A California case, *Niles* v. *City of San Rafael,* 42 Cal. App. 3d 230, 116 Cal. Rptr. 733 (1974), demonstrates how important it is to adhere to departmental policies and procedures in the emergency department of a general hospital.

The case involved an 11-year-old boy. The child suffered a head injury in the schoolyard and was brought to the emergency room of the defendant hospital by his father. The nurses, intern, and resident physician on duty all agreed the boy needed to be admitted for observation. An employee of the admitting office erroneously told the intern that the child could not be admitted because he was not being treated by a physician with hospital staff privileges. The intern, with the resident, then sought the help of the physician-director of the hospital's pediatric outpatient clinic to have the boy admitted. The director, without even seeing the child, discharged him from care. The director thus compounded the admitting clerk's error.

The director instructed the boy's father to watch the child for pupil dilation and to be sure the child could be roused when sleeping. These instructions were also contrary to emergency room policy because discharge policies for this kind of injury were clearly written in the hospital. Before a youngster with a possible head injury was to be released from the emergency room, the policy stipulated that the parents were to be given a sheet listing signs and symptoms, with the warning to return the child to the emergency room if any of these signs or symptoms appeared. Not only was this sheet not given to the father, but five of the signs and symptoms were present when the child was released.

The results were disastrous. Because treatment was delayed, the child suffered intracranial bleeding and was totally disabled. He suffers complete paralysis from the neck down, except for slight movement of the right hand and foot. He sees and hears well but is mute. The brain damage, at this time, appears to be irreparable.

From this case, one can readily see the importance of following established policies. During the course of the trial, an expert witness for the plaintiff testified that permanent damage could have been avoided had the child been treated immediately. No testimony was offered by the defendant hospital and physician to show circumstances explaining the errors made. In this case, those errors resulted in a paralyzed child and a $4 million judgment against the hospital and the physician-director of the pediatric outpatient clinic.

Chapter 4

Issues of Consent

Another part of the admission process that raises legal questions concerns consent to treatment. This chapter will explore the nature of consent, the meaning of informed consent, the right of a patient to refuse or withdraw consent, implied consent, and consent in a true emergency. We will also discuss consent forms and the law in regard to minors and people who are mentally incompetent.

THE NATURE OF CONSENT: GENERAL PRINCIPLES

Consent to treatment is necessary because the intentional touching of a person for the purpose of health, without his or her consent, is legally a battery. Thus, barring an emergency or a court order that compels treatment, consent to treatment is always needed. Whether or not the treatment is performed willfully, or whether or not negligence is involved, does not change the fact that the person who renders treatment without consent is legally liable for battery.

Although assault and battery charges are frequently criminal charges brought by the state in a criminal court, these charges may also be brought by a plaintiff-patient as civil charges in a civil court against anyone who authorized or performed the treatment.

Consent, in the law, applies only to acts that are legal. Therefore, a person cannot consent to an illegal act. Prior to 1973 a woman could not legally consent to an abortion if that treatment or act was illegal in the state in which she resided.

In an emergency situation, treatment to preserve life or prevent permanent bodily damage may be administered without first obtaining consent from the patient. This is because the law implies consent due to the emergency nature of the situation.

Under the law, any person who is mentally competent to understand the significance of her or his acts is able to either consent to or refuse treatment. A person who has not reached the age of majority is not legally able to consent to or refuse treatment. An individual who is not a minor but who is intoxicated, or under the influence of medication, or is not mentally competent to understand the consequences of his or her acts is also not legally capable of consenting to or refusing treatment.

Consent, in order to be legally valid, must be informed consent. The requirement for informed consent is met when the individual is given enough information to understand to what he or she is consenting. "Enough information" implies information that allows the patient to choose among treatments—that is, to opt for one treatment while electing to refuse others.

Consent to treatment must also be specific; general consent is invalid because it does not meet the test of informed consent. Consent to treatment should thus be obtained for *each* treatment the person is receiving.

If consent is being sought for medical treatment such as surgery, it is the legal duty of the surgeon to obtain the patient's consent. The duty cannot legally be delegated by the surgeon to another health practitioner. Similarly, if consent is sought for a nursing treatment, the consent must be obtained by a nurse and cannot legally be delegated to a health practitioner in another discipline.

In the law, oral consent is just as valid as written consent. However, for purposes of documentation and to avoid litigation, written consent is clearly preferable.

Once given, consent may legally be withdrawn or revoked at any time. The withdrawal may be in oral or written form; however, as mentioned in the discussion on the giving of consent, withdrawal in writing is certainly preferable to oral withdrawal.

Specific consent, once given, cannot be extended beyond that to which the patient originally consented. Thus if the patient has given specific consent to a laparoscopy, that consent is legally valid only for that procedure. It cannot be extended to allow a hysterectomy. This extension of consent rule does not apply in the case of an emergency—that is, where the treatment is necessary to preserve life or prevent permanent bodily damage.

The general principles outlined above govern consent to treatment and are well established in the courts. A careful look at the decisions of the courts on the issue of consent may well lead one to believe that consistency is not always practiced. This apparent inconsistency is attributable to the facts involved in each individual case.

The remainder of this chapter will concentrate on a detailed explanation of the principles sketched in this section. At the end of this discussion the reader should recognize the importance of having hospital administrators, nurses, physicians, and other health personnel seek a court order when consent to treatment is refused on the grounds of religious or other convictions. The reader will also learn how court cases have dealt with consent to treatment in emergency versus nonemergency situations.

INFORMED CONSENT IN MEDICAL PROCEDURES

The conclusions that can be drawn from court rulings on the principles of consent are these:

- A competent person who has reached the age of majority will almost always be granted the right to accept or refuse treatment *if* she or he has no minor children to whom is owed a duty of parental care.

- An adult parent of minor children or person with other family responsibilities almost invariably will be compelled to undertake unwanted but life-preserving treatment.

- In the case of minors, there has been no case where a court allowed the parents or legal guardians of a child to refuse treatment for the child where that treatment was aimed at preserving or prolonging the child's life.

There are two important points to understand about consent. The first is that in some states liability can attach even if the treatment aided the patient's condition, *if* the procedure was done without the patient's consent. A second point is that in an emergency consent is implied, and thus treatment should not be delayed in order to obtain consent.

A case in point is *Cooper* v. *Roberts,* 220 Pa. Super. 260, 286 A. 2d 647 (1971), a minority view at the time. A patient was admitted to a hospital for tests and studies of a hiatal hernia. As no emergency was involved, consent was obtained. The patient signed a blanket consent form authorizing procedures her doctor found necessary and advisable. The attending physician and the hospital radiologist agreed that a gastroscopic examination was needed. The patient was not informed of any collateral risks. During the procedure, her stomach was punctured. The patient sued, arguing that the physician had not informed her of the risks of the procedure and of the available alternatives.

Although the patient was not successful in trial court, judgment having been denied, she successfully appealed to the Superior Court in Pennsylvania and a new trial was held. The court ruled that the law in the Commonwealth of Pennsylvania is that where a patient is mentally and physically able to consult about his condition, in the absence of an emergency, that patient's "informed consent" is a prerequisite to a surgical operation by his or her physician. An operation without such informed consent is a technical assault, making the physician liable for any injuries resulting from the invasion, regardless of whether or not the treatment was negligently administered.

The physician is bound to disclose only those risks which a reasonable person would consider material to the decision of whether or not to undergo treatment. The test is *not* the amount of disclosure that would have been made by a reasonable practitioner, but rather whether the doctor disclosed facts, risks, and alternatives that would have been considered significant to a reasonable person faced with making such a decision. By so framing the test, the court eliminated the need of having other practitioners offer expert testimony on what disclosures other physicians make in obtaining consent. The test, framed in the terms of a reasonable person making a decision, was workable for a jury.

The jury returned a judgment for the plaintiff-patient, stressing that a patient has a right to know all the material facts pertaining to proposed treatment.

In a 1972 California case, *Cobbs* v. *Grant,* 104 Cal. Rptr. 505, 502 P. 2d 1, the court stated four guiding principles on consent. They are: (1)   the knowledge of physician and patient are not in parity; (2)   the adult patient of sound mind has the right to determine whether or not he will submit to lawful medical treatment; (3)   the patient's consent must be informed consent; and (4)   as regards medical information, the patient is dependent on the physician for the information on which to base a decision, raising an obligation on the physician. Therefore, a physician must develop "all information relevant to a meaningful decisional process" (*Cobbs* v. *Grant,* 104 Cal Rptr 505, 513).

The facts in this case revealed that a surgical procedure had been performed for an intractable peptic duodenal ulcer. The physician explained the nature of the operation but did not discuss the dangers inherent in surgery. The ulcer disappeared following the surgery, but during the surgery an artery at the hilum of the spleen was severed, causing internal bleeding. On discovering this nine days later, the physician removed the patient's spleen. The risk of such injury is five percent. Further complications, including a gastric ulcer, later developed. The physician then had to remove half of the patient's stomach to reduce its acid-producing capacity. Premature absorption of a suture caused bleeding, another risk, which necessitated rehospitalization.

The court in *Cobbs* rejected the majority rule that the physician's duty to inform a patient is judged by the prevailing standards of the medical community. The court held that the physician-defendant had the duty to make reasonable disclosure to the patient of the choices available with respect to a proposed therapy and of the inherent and potential dangers of each therapy. Since the patient's right of self-decision is the measure of the doctor's duty to inform, reasonable disclosure means that all perils material to the patient's decision must be divulged. There must, however, be a causal relationship between the failure to inform and the patient's injury. If the patient would have consented to the procedure given all the material information, then there is no liability.

According to the court, the question must be resolved by the test of what a prudent person in the patient's position would have decided if adequately informed of all significant perils. Thus the failure to adequately inform is grounds for negligence, according to *Cobbs* v. *Grant.*

An earlier Florida case, *Bowers* v. *Talmadge,* 159 So. 2d. 888 (Dist. Ct. of App. of Fla., 1963) dealt with this same issue in a different way. In this case, neurosurgeons gave expert testimony to show that it was customary to inform those who had to make a decision for a specific procedure that the operation was dangerous. The defendant-physician had not so informed the parents of the child-patient, and so the decision over whether the consent was informed and legally valid was left for the jury to determine.

The injured plaintiff was a child. Because the child had a number of visual complaints—such as seeing things, etc.—his parents took him to a neurosurgeon recommended by the boy's physician. Because the neurosurgeon was not sure whether the problem was emotional or organic, the physician-defendant suggested an arteriogram (an exploratory surgical procedure) rather than psychiatric treatment.

The court pointed out that no emergency existed requiring the procedure. Indeed, the court stated that the arteriogram was optional and merely one alternative to treatment. The court emphasized an arteriogram *is* a dangerous procedure, with a three percent known number of cases resulting in death, paralysis, or other injury. In this case the plaintiff-child did suffer partial paralysis as a result of the arteriogram.

The court decided, on appeal, that there had been conflicting evidence as to whether informed consent for the arteriogram had been obtained from the parents. The court stated that the parents' consent had to have been obtained, citing earlier court cases as precedent for this rule. The court also pointed out that a consent given without knowing the dangers and the degrees of danger is not a valid consent because it does not represent a choice. The physician-defendant was obligated to adequately inform the parents of the possible dangers, and not to minimize those dangers. The defense had shown no grounds for an exception to that rule.

The parents did present evidence that the neurosurgeon did not inform them of the dangers. In addition, the court followed the majority rule of the customary behavior of practitioners, and the parents had testimony by neurosurgeons that it *was* customary to inform the decision makers that an arteriogram is a dangerous procedure. The judgment for the physician-defendant was reversed, and the parents won the right to a new trial.

In *Coppage* v. *Gamble*, 324 So. 2d 21 (1976), a Louisiana court considered the question of consent *implied* from voluntary submission to treatment. The facts in this case reveal that the plaintiff presented himself to the podiatrist-defendant with a history of foot problems and acute pain in the left foot. After examining the patient the podiatrist recommended surgery. Although the surgery was performed successfully in a hospital, the podiatrist had failed to obtain written authorization for the surgery. The patient sued both the podiatrist and the hospital for doing unnecessary surgery and for failing to obtain the patient's consent for removal of a part of the metatarsal bone.

Both in the lower court and on appeal, the judicial decision was that the podiatrist had adequately informed the patient of his condition. The podiatrist introduced into evidence rough drawings of the proposed surgery, sketched in his office as he explained the operation to the patient. The court held for the podiatrist on the ground that *either* the patient had *orally* agreed or had voluntarily submitted to treatment by admitting himself for surgery. The court labeled this situation implied consent, although that appears to be a misnomer. Nevertheless, the podiatrist could have easily saved himself the anguish of a lawsuit by obtaining written consent to the precise surgical procedure.

The above cases dealt with informed consent as it relates to physicians. Although the rules can vary from state to state, the basic rule is one of either full or reasonable disclosure. Reasonable disclosure allows that there need not be a discussion of relatively minor dangers that occur so infrequently as to be remote possibilities.

NURSES AND INFORMED CONSENT

In contrast to medical procedures, where there is a wealth of case law, there is relatively little authority on the duty of hospital employees to inform, and little on the duty of nurses to obtain informed consent for nursing procedures.

The prudent nurse should keep in mind the example of physicians and informed consent, and extend the logic of these court rulings to her own practice. Certainly nurses have a professional duty to do what is best for their patients and render safe care. The nurse should not conceal information about nursing procedures when that information would be necessary in helping a reasonably prudent person decide whether to accept or refuse the treatment.

In today's expanded role for nurses, many nurses, especially nurse practitioners, provide primary care. In these situations, consent should clearly be obtained before the nursing procedures and treatments are administered.

There is little guidance as to how much information nurses must divulge to obtain informed consent. Future years should provide court rulings and other authority. In the interim, nurses should watch current court rulings on informed consent and use these as a guide.

THE TRUE EMERGENCY

In a true emergency, consent to treatment is implied. That is, the law reasons that had the patient been able to give consent, he or she certainly would have done so.

The true emergency is generally defined as one in which treatment is required to prevent death—that is, to preserve life or prevent permanent bodily harm. The rationale is that to delay treatment in order to obtain consent could result in greater harm or injury.

An old Michigan case shows how the courts treat the issue of consent in an emergency situation. In *Luka* v. *Lowrie,* 171 Mich. 122, 136 N.W. 1106 (1912), the Superior Court of Michigan held that the emergency justified an operation without consent. In this case the facts reveal that a 15-year-old boy suffered a crushing injury to his foot from a train car while crossing railroad tracks. Four hospital physicians and a surgeon agreed that amputation was necessary to save the child's life. The court, in holding for the defendant-physician, reasoned that had the parents been present to give consent, they would have.

In some situations where parents refuse to give consent for treatment considered life-saving or life-prolonging, the court will compel parents to allow treatment for the child. The theory in this situation is that the state is the protector of all persons unable to protect themselves. Thus when the natural parents or legal guardians are unfit, the state may act in the child's best interests.

As stated in *Lowrie,* the threat to life or health must be immediate to constitute an emergency. Thus if delay would increase the hazards to the patient, then treatment can be undertaken without consent. However, if treatment may be medically advisable, but delay would not increase the hazards, treatment should not be initiated.

For an example of a court ruling on this principle, one could look at *Zoski* v. *Gaines,* 271 Mich. 1, 260 N.W. 99 (1935). In this case the surgeon was held liable by the court for removing the allegedly infected tonsils of a minor without first having obtained parental consent. The court reasoned that no immediate necessity had been shown for removing the tonsils at that time. Therefore, consent should have been obtained before the surgical procedure.

Every effort should be made to document the need for treatment without consent. It must be shown that there was actually an immediate threat to life or health. Thus, in a hospital emergency room, the chart or record should document that consultation took place before the procedure was begun. The record should clearly specify the nature of the threat to life or health, its immediacy, and its magnitude. Additionally, the record should document that it was impossible to obtain consent and why it was impossible. The hospital, through its employees, then need not obtain consent in the case of an emergency. The law implies consent because of the emergency.

The emergency *only* should be treated. That is, treatment that goes *beyond* that needed for the emergency condition cannot be given.

A physician should make the determination that immediate treatment is needed as soon as the patient is brought to the emergency room, to prevent a worsening of the patient's condition. The scope of the emergency needs to be determined also. Treatment may consist of temporary medical care, such as arresting hemorrhage, or may include surgical procedures.

Although no legal ruling requires consultation, and in some emergencies time alone may preclude a consultation, one should be sought whenever possible to confirm the existence of an emergency. The consultant's opinion should be documented.

Hospitals should adapt and disseminate to their employees clearly written policies on consent for treatment. The policies should cover not only the matter of obtaining consent, but also refusal and withdrawal of consent. The policies should also include advice on situations involving minors and others unable to give valid consent.

A hospital's liability for providing treatment without consent is based on either respondeat superior or the duty of the hospital to prevent injury to patients committed by third parties. A hospital faces liability whenever someone on its staff commits a battery. Under the doctrine of respondeat superior, the hospital, as employer, must respond and account for the actions of its employees. Hospital liability can be predicated on a breach of the duty to obtain consent for routine procedures such as laboratory tests. It can also be based on the hospital's duty to obtain consent for procedures ordered by a patient's private physician but performed by hospital employees (such as intravenous feedings). Liability can also be predicated on a breach of the hospital's duty to monitor the physician-employees of the hospital as well as the private physicians who are allowed to use the facility.

In *Schwartz* v. *Boston Hospital for Women*, 422 F. Supp. 53 (S.D.N.Y., 1976), a patient sued a hospital arguing that the hospital had reason to know or believe that her doctor's procedures were clearly contraindicated by normal practice. The patient charged that the curettage that was performed on her following a Cesarean section was done without her consent and was performed not for her own personal reasons but to further an ongoing research study into maternal-infant health problems in diabetic pregnancies. This procedure, the patient claimed, was medically contraindicated and, in fact, caused her subsequent infection and sterility. In denying the hospital's motion for summary judgment, the court recognized that the medical staff of a hospital has a duty to monitor actions of its physicians, especially those physicians who are paid by the hospital to perform medical duties. The duty to monitor, the court found, includes ensuring that physicians have secured all necessary consents from any patients participating in an experimental study and stopping those procedures that seem clearly inconsistent with good practice.

CONSENT FORMS

Although oral consent is legally valid, written consent is preferable because it has the advantage of being easier to prove. To be legally effective a written consent (1)   must be signed voluntarily, (2)   must show that the procedure performed was the one to which consent was given, and (3)   must show that the person giving the consent understood the nature of the procedure, the risks involved, and the probable consequences.

A general consent form, signed on admission to a hospital and worded to permit a physician to perform any medical or surgical procedure in the patient's best interest, at the discretion of the physician, is legally invalid. It is as if the patient signs no consent form at all. In both situations, were a court suit filed, testimony would be needed to show what the patient actually knew of the situation. A jury would have to listen to all the testimony given and determine whom to believe.

For example, in *Rogers* v. *Lumbermens Mutual Casualty Co.,* 119 So. 2d 649 (La. Sup. Ct., 1960), a form signed by the patient stating that her physician(s) in charge were authorized to administer such treatment, and the surgeon such anesthetics, as they found necessary to perform the operation that was advisable in her treatment was not effective because it failed to designate the exact nature of the operation authorized. The plaintiff-patient had considerable evidence to show that she was ignorant of any possibility that her reproductive organs would be removed during her appendectomy. The surgeon involved testified that there was no emergency and that he removed the reproductive organs as a precautionary measure. Moreover, the patient's husband, her married daughter, and her son-in-law were nearby in the hospital during the operation, and the court felt that they could have been contacted to obtain consent.

The General Consent Form and the Special Consent Form

The best approach seems to be to have a patient sign two consent forms: a general consent form (signed in the admitting office) and a special consent form. The general consent form may seem unnecessary insofar as patients who voluntarily admit themselves to a hospital could be seen as implying consent for hospital services such as tests, procedures, and examinations. However, the general consent form signed on admission does serve as documentation of voluntary admission and general authorization. During admission the patient should also be informed of the hospital rules and policies designed for the safety and care of patients.

A special consent form should be signed by the patient before individual, specific procedures are performed—that is, those other than routine hospital procedures. Completion of the special consent form should not take place in the hospital's admitting office. The task of providing the necessary information to patients and answering their questions requires a knowledge of medicine that only a physician has. If a procedure that normally calls for special consent is scheduled to be performed very soon after admission, it may be possible for the physician to provide the information and obtain the patient's consent prior to admission, in the physician's office.

Use of the special consent form presupposes a pattern for disclosure in the conversations between the physician and the patient, a pattern that ensures that necessary matters are covered. Without a disclosure pattern that provides the patient with the necessary information, the form offers few benefits. A full disclosure that is documented on the form provides protection from possible liability.

The special consent form thus shows that the patient understands the specific treatment to be undertaken. In general, this form should be signed before any type of surgery is performed, before any type of anesthesia is used, and for nonsurgical procedures involving more than a slight risk of harm or a risk of change in the patient's body structure. More specifically, a signed special consent form should be obtained before any of the following procedures are carried out:

- Major or minor surgery that involves an entry into the body either through an incision or through one of the natural body openings

- All procedures in which anesthesia is used, regardless of whether an entry into the body is involved

- Nonsurgical procedures involving more than a slight risk of harm to the patient, or involving the risk of a change in the patient's body structure. Such procedures would include, but are not limited to, diagnostic procedures such as myelograms, arteriograms, and pyelograms.

- Procedures involving the use of cobalt and x-ray therapy

- Electroshock therapy

- Experimental procedures

- All other procedures that the medical staff determines require a specific explanation to the patient. Any doubts as to the necessity of obtaining a special consent from the patient should be resolved in favor of obtaining the consent.

For consent forms, either general or special, it is unnecessary to have a signature by a witness to make the consent effective. The patient's signature alone is adequate. There is, however, no rule against providing for the signature of a witness, and indeed it is probably advisable to have one witness who can attest that the patient's signature is genuine.

The special consent form should include the exact date and time that consent is obtained. This is important because it is documented evidence that consent was obtained at a time that the patient was not under preoperative medication and therefore was competent to consent. It is best to explain the procedure requiring consent while the patient is neither in pain nor drugged. The special consent should be obtained shortly before the procedure. If more than a few days lapse between the patient's signed consent and the performance of the procedure, it is advisable to obtain another signed consent form.

There should be space in the form for an explanation of the condition to be treated and the need to treat that condition. Courts have found it easier to infer that a patient has consented to all reasonable steps to correct a condition if this is clearly stated in the consent form. The description should be written in plain language, easily understood by the average person. If the patient does not read English, the form should provide space showing that the explanation was made in the patient's language, and the name of the translator should appear on the form. The name of the physician obtaining consent for the procedure should also appear on the form.

If a series of procedures is planned over a period of time, the consent form should reflect this. If not, a new form should be signed by the patient for each new procedure.

Possible risks and consequences of the procedure should be included in the special consent form. Courts have found lack of consent when consequences and risks that commonly follow a procedure were not explained to a patient.

The form should include permission for the physician to use anesthesia, and the specific anesthesia to be used should be identified. In addition, any photographs should be authorized before they are taken. This will preclude the patient from later bringing suit for invasion of privacy.

The hospital should be authorized to keep tissues, and this should be provided for in the special consent form.

The form should also include a statement that no guarantee has been promised as to cure.

Finally, the form should include a statement that the patient is aware that additional questions, if any, can be asked *after* signing the form, but that no additional questions exist at the time the form is signed. This shows that enough information has been given.

Refusal to Consent

Clearly, a minor, one who is not conscious, or one who is mentally incompetent cannot legally give consent.

If a patient refuses to sign a consent form in total or refuses to agree to any segment of it, this must be noted in the patient's record and respected. If a patient refuses to consent to a procedure, a release form should be completed and added to the patient's record to protect against liability for not performing the procedure. Should the patient refuse to sign the release form, this refusal should be recorded in the patient's record.

In a true emergency, where treatment must be initiated in order to prevent death or permanent bodily injury, one should not delay treatment in order to obtain the patient's signed consent form. However, many emergency room cases are not of this nature, and for these a consent form should be signed by the patient. In nonemergency cases where it is impossible to obtain written consent, as in the case of a minor with parents in another location, a telegram or monitored phone call would be the best alternative.

A consent form cannot be written to constitute a general release of the physician or hospital from liability. In *Belshaw* v. *Feinstein,* 258 Cal. App. 2d 420, 65, Cal. Rptr. 788 (1968), the patient and his wife executed written releases before the first step of the operational procedure, and again before the second operative procedure. These were to release the physician and hospital from liability due to any and all untoward risks or complications resulting from the surgical procedures. The court found these exculpatory agreements void as against public policy. The court held that a provision releasing one from liability for future negligence may stand only if it does not involve the public interest.

Even in an emergency, a patient has the legal right to refuse treatment. A conscious adult who is mentally competent has the right to refuse medical treatment, even when the best medical opinion deems that treatment necessary to save the patient's life. In all the cases that establish and support the rule that an emergency gives a physician a privilege to treat a patient without consent, the patient was incapable of manifesting a refusal to consent, either because of unconsciousness, or because of lack of capacity, such as minority. No case has applied the emergency rule in the face of a competent patient's express refusal to consent.

The decision to save the patient's life in the face of an express prohibition by the patient is a humanitarian one, but may not be supported by the law. Legally, the patient's refusal is to be respected and, thus, there is a risk of liability for proceeding in the face of the refusal. Even if the procedure is performed skillfully, the patient's right to be secure in his or her person has been violated, and the patient may seek damages for the unauthorized treatment. It is doubtful that the legal situation is changed if, after the patient's refusal, the physician waits until the patient lapses into unconsciousness and then commences treatment, justifying action on the existence of an emergency. Although the physician's motivation would be understandable, the doctor's desire to preserve life may not outweigh a person's right to control his or her destiny and be the sole determinator of what should be done to his or her body.

Courts have been drawn into the difficult questions inherent in a patient's refusal of treatment. They have also been concerned with the effect of refusal of treatment by a close relative of the patient. In a New York case, *Collins* v. *Davis*, 44 N.Y. Misc. 2d 622, 254 N.Y.S. 2d 666 (Sup. Ct. Nassau County, 1964), where the patient was unconscious and unable to either refuse or give consent, his spouse refused to authorize surgical treatment. The court stated that it was convinced by the physicians' affidavits and by the hospital records that the patient would die unless the operation was performed and therefore authorized treatment. The court pointed out that the physicians who were attending the patient should not be exposed to liability for either an unauthorized procedure (if they proceeded with treatment) or for malpractice (if necessary treatment was not given). The court held that it would make the decision and insulate the physicians from those liability risks.

MINORS

Minors lack legal competence to consent to treatment, and authorization is required from the parents or legal guardian. Thus a consent form signed by a minor would not be effective.

There are exceptions to this general rule. An emergency situation is the most important exception. Parental consent is implied in situations that call for immediate action to preserve a life or prevent permanent bodily harm—that is, in cases of true emergency.

Another exception applies in the case of a minor who is married or legally emancipated. Every state and the District of Columbia have defined the age of majority within their borders. The age of majority in most states is 18 years.

In Pennsylvania and Mississippi it is 21 years. In Alabama, Alaska, Nebraska, and Wyoming it is 19 years. Below that age, individuals are legally minors and lack capacity to consent to or refuse treatment.

Legally, emancipation of a minor means that the parents have surrendered entirely their right to care, custody, and earnings of the minor child; the parents have renounced their parental duties and responsibilities. Emancipation is generally by agreement of the parents and child, though it may be by court decision. The emancipation may be expressed in writing or may be implied from conduct. Emancipation implies that the child is able to take care of himself or herself. The child may leave the parental home, make his or her own living, receive his or her own wages, and spend these wages as he or she pleases.

Usually, but not invariably, emancipation does not take place before the child is 16 years old. Because emancipated minors do not usually carry identification as such, emergency room personnel should look for evidence of an address separate from the parents, evidence of a job, or other indications of self-support. Emancipation obligates the minor to pay the cost of health care.

Most states recognize some form of emancipation of minors. In addition to emancipation as defined above, marriage of a minor is seen as emancipation. In Pennsylvania, all minors who are high school graduates or are parents or are pregnant are legally emancipated. Pennsylvania is, however, an exception to the general rule.

The mature minor is a relatively new concept, applicable to youths who are sufficiently mature and intelligent to understand the nature and consequences of a treatment that is for their benefit. Mature minors are to be distinguished from those minors who lack maturity, usually, but not always, by reason of age. Courts have recognized mature minors in several decisions, often in situations where parents and child differ on the choice of treatment. For example, a minor who wants birth control devices because he or she fully understands their importance to sexual activity, demonstrates the ability to make a mature decision. Similarly, where minors elect to have an abortion because they recognize and appreciate their incapacity to be parents, they show the ability to understand the nature and consequences of their decisions. Where the parents have differed with the child's choice of treatment, the courts have upheld the minor's decision by invoking the concept of the mature minor.

The last exception is the statutory exception allowing minors to consent to treatment for venereal disease, drug abuse, and pregnancy-related care. All states have enacted legislation in these areas to dispense with the requirement of parental consent for minors.

All in all, the judicial trend on questions of minors consenting to treatment has been to uphold the rights of minors. It would seem that the safest course would be to obtain consent from the parents of all young minors. In the case of teen-agers, it is probably best to obtain consent from the minor, if he or she is able to understand the nature of the consent, but also obtain the consent of the parent or legal guardian.

If a child is a minor attending college, away from home, school administrators may sign consent forms by designation of the parents. In this case, the teen-age minor should also be asked to sign the consent form.

If the patient has reached the age of majority and is competent, it may be held to be an invasion of the patient's right of privacy to inform the spouse, parent, or guardian.

Where the parents refuse to consent to treatment for a minor child, the courts must be petitioned for a court order mandating treatment.

A married minor's consent to treatment for his or her child would appear to be effective where emancipation through marriage is recognized or where the maturity of the individual minor is considered.

In a Pennsylvania case, *In re Green,* 292 A. 2d 387 (1972), the Director of the State Hospital for Crippled Children sought a judicial declaration, under Pennsylvania law, that Ricardo Green, 17, was a neglected child. The child had suffered two attacks of poliomyelitis which left him with a 94 percent curvature of the spine. The mother, a Jehovah's Witness, consented to surgery to alleviate the curvature, but the consent was given on the condition that there be no blood transfusions on religious grounds.

Under the statute, a neglected child is one "whose parent—neglects or refuses to provide proper or necessary medical or surgical care" [The Juvenile Court Law, Act of June 2, 1933, P.L. 1433, Sec. 1(5) (c), as amended 11 P.S. Sec. 243(5) (6) (c)]. The question for the court was whether the state could interfere with a parent's control over his or her child in order to enhance the child's well-being, when the child's life is in no immediate danger and when the state's intrusion conflicts with the parent's religious beliefs. The court held that the state did not have an interest of sufficient magnitude to outweigh a parent's religious belief when the child's life is not *immediately imperiled* by his physical condition. The court remanded the case for an evidentiary hearing to determine the child's wishes.

This case shows how much importance the court placed on the lack of emergency in the situation. Three judges dissented; they felt the court should intervene since there was a substantial threat to the child's well-being and health, and also because they felt the child was too dependent on his parents to make an independent decision.

WITHDRAWAL OF CONSENT

Consent may be withdrawn at any time after consent has been given. The patient has the absolute legal right to revoke or withdraw consent. As with the consent itself, oral withdrawal is just as legally effective as written withdrawal. However, for purposes of evidence and documentation, it is preferable to have withdrawal of consent in writing. Even though the consent for the treatment or procedure was written, an oral withdrawal of consent is legally valid. Once the consent is withdrawn, orally or in writing, performing the procedure or treatment amounts to a legal battery.

In the case of surgery, the consent form may be revoked by a patient at any time prior to preoperative medication. Providing the patient is competent and clearly understands the consequences of withdrawing or revoking consent, it is legally effective for the patient to revoke the original consent.

MORE ON REFUSAL OF CONSENT

Patients have the absolute legal right to refuse to consent to treatment. When health practitioners believe treatment is essential, but the patient refuses to consent—whether because of religious convictions or other reasons, a court order should be sought.

This is true in emergency and nonemergency situations. A competent patient's refusal must be honored, whether the refusal is grounded on doubt that the procedure will be effective or successful, concern about the results of the procedure, lack of confidence in the physician or other health professionals who recommend the treatment or procedure, religious convictions, fear, or mere whim.

In *Erickson* v. *Dilgard,* 44 Misc. 2d 27, 252 N.Y.S. 2d 705 (1962), the hospital sought court authorization for a blood transfusion for a patient who refused it. The patient had been admitted to the hospital with a diagnosis of upper gastrointestinal bleeding. The patient was willing to have surgery but refused a blood transfusion. The hospital's contention was that the patient would have little chance of recovery without the blood.

Testimony showed that the patient was completely competent and capable of making decisions on his own behalf, that he understood the increased risk of having the operation without the transfusion, and that the refusal of a transfusion represented the patient's calculated decision.

The court stated that it is always a question of judgment whether the medical decision is correct, and held that the individual who is the subject of a medical decision should have the final say. The court denied the hospital's application to authorize the administration of a blood transfusion and upheld the patient's right of refusal.

In a similar case in Illinois, the court also held that a competent adult who did not have minor children had the right to refuse a blood transfusion that was against her religious beliefs. *In re Brooks Estate,* 32 Ill. 2d 361, 205 N.E. 2d 435 (1965), the patient and her husband had executed documents releasing the doctor and hospital from civil liability.

But there are times when a court finds a compelling state interest that justifies interference with a person's religious beliefs. At about the time the previous cases were decided, a Washington, D.C. court, in a leading case, *Application of the President and Directors of Georgetown College, Inc.,* 331 F 2d 1000 (D.C. Cir., 1964), ordered a blood transfusion for a patient who had refused it. Here the court reasoned that the woman had a duty to her infant child that overrode her right to refuse.

In *In re Osborne,* 294 A. 2d 372 (D.C. Ct. App., 1972), the court expressed the state's interest in the welfare of the children of patients who refuse blood transfusions on religious grounds. In this case the patient had made financial provisions for his two minor children so they would not become wards of the state if he expired, and he had a large family that was willing to care for the children. Additionally, the patient, with full understanding, had executed a statement refusing the transfusion and releasing the hospital from liability. The court upheld the patient's right to refuse the transfusion. The patient recovered without the transfusion and was released from the hospital.

These and similar rulings clearly support two conclusions: (1) a competent adult without minor children almost invariably will be granted the right, by the courts, to accept or refuse treatment; and (2) a competent adult with minor children or other major family responsibilities will often be compelled by the courts to undergo unwanted but life-saving treatment.

No case has been found where a court permitted parents or guardians to refuse treatment for a minor where the treatment was intended to preserve or prolong the child's life. Thus hospital personnel should request a court order whenever a patient refuses, for whatever reasons, to consent to life-saving treatment.

MENTAL INCOMPETENCE

Since consent must be voluntary and must be based on a comprehension of the nature of the procedure or treatment, an individual who is mentally incompetent cannot legally give consent. For an individual who has been declared legally incompetent in a judicial proceeding, it is necessary to obtain the consent of the patient's legal guardian. When this is not possible, a court order should be sought.

Patient consent obtained from one who is generally unable to comprehend information will be treated by the courts as invalid. For purposes of consent, competency is defined as an ability to understand the nature and consequences of that to which one is asked to consent. As such, mental incompetency is not limited to those who have been declared legally incompetent. It includes those who, in the opinion of the attending physician, are either permanently (e.g., mentally deficient, senile) or temporarily (e.g., head injury, alcohol or drug abuse) incapable of giving consent.

If a guardian or conservator "of the person" has been appointed, said guardian or conservator must consent to treatment. However, when the patient explicitly refuses such treatment, the physician should require that the guardian or conservator obtain specific court authorization before proceeding. Prior to providing treatment, a certified copy of the official letters of guardianship or conservatorship should be obtained, placed in, and made part of the patient's permanent medical record.

In a situation where emergency treatment is not indicated, if a guardian or conservator has not been court-appointed, and the attending physician is of the opinion that the patient is either temporarily or permanently incompetent, treatment should be delayed until either the patient regains competency or a guardian or conservator has been appointed. If obtaining a court-appointed guardian or conservator is not possible, a court must be asked for permission to perform the treatment or procedure.

A person who is mentally ill should have the same right to choose or refuse treatment as the person who is physically ill, so long as the mental illness does not render the person incompetent to choose. In *Bell* v. *Wayne County General Hospital at Eloise,* 384 F. Supp. 1085 (E.D. Mich., 1974), the court held that treatment may not be given to a person allegedly mentally ill until a court proceeding has finally adjudicated that individual mentally ill, unless the person voluntarily consents to treatment or the treatment is necessary to prevent physical self-harm or harm to others (as clearly demonstrated by acts of the patient or other objective criteria).

Where there is doubt as to a patient's competency to consent, but the patient has not been declared legally incompetent, the consent of the nearest relative should be sought. If the patient is unable to consent, the spouse is the first person from whom to seek consent. However, if the patient is mentally competent to give consent, the consent of the spouse without the consent of the competent patient would be invalid. Competent patients must give their own consent.

Chapter 5

Patient Transfers

As we have seen in the discussion in Chapter 3 of admission policies and problems, when a hospital undertakes to treat a person, it must not act unreasonably in removing or in having that person removed from the premises. The law requires that a patient be kept in the hospital and that treatment be continued if it is foreseeable that the patient's condition would be aggravated or the risk of danger increased by removal.

It is not necessary, however, for a hospital to keep a patient until he or she is cured. A patient may be transferred to another hospital so long as the risk of harm to the patient resulting from the transfer is not unreasonable. Thus in *Willis* v. *Western Hospital Association,* 67 Idaho 435, 182 P. 2d 950 (1947), the removal of a patient to a hospital for the insane, after a judicial order for commitment was obtained, was not improper in the absence of a showing that the transfer resulted in or hastened the death of the patient.

It should be noted that in certain circumstances there may be a duty to transfer the patient to another hospital after emergency treatment, if the first hospital does not have the proper facilities and equipment for the patient's continued care. In *Carrasco* v. *Bankoff,* 220 Cal. App. 230, 33 Cal Rptr. 673 (1963), liability was imposed on the hospital which, although not equipped to treat serious burns, had retained a patient with third-degree burns for 53 days before transfer to a hospital that had appropriate treatment facilities. Damages were awarded for the additional hospitalization and treatment, and for the permanent scars and deformities that were largely a result of the delay in transferring the patient to a hospital that could render adequate care.

In the transfer of a psychiatric patient, the law imposes a duty to exercise reasonable care in regard to the patient, recognizing the mental condition and status of the patient, if known. Thus it is important to take necessary and adequate precautions to restrain the patient for self-protection and the protection of the staff. This is even more important if the patient displays aggressiveness. The patient must be protected from self-inflicted injury, and the staff accompanying the patient in a transfer must be protected from the patient's potentially dangerous behavior.

In preparing records to accompany the transferred patient, it is essential to prepare complete and accurate documentation. This would include, of course, a complete medical history.

EXTERNAL STANDARDS ON TRANSFERRALS

In 1972, following a three-year study by the American Hospital Association's board of trustees and four consumer representatives, the AHA Bill of Rights was approved as a national policy statement. Most hospitals adopted this statement of patients' rights. The AHA Bill of Rights addresses 12 rights of patients. One of these, Right No. 7, has to do with the patient who is transferred. It reads:

> The patient has the right to expect that within its capacity a hospital must make reasonable response to the request of a patient for services. The hospital must provide evaluation, service, and/or referral as indicated by the urgency of the case. When medically permissible, a patient may be transferred to another facility only after he has received complete information and explanation concerning the needs for and alternatives to such a transfer. The institution to which the patient is to be transferred must first have accepted the patient for transfer.[1]

The Joint Commission on Accreditation of Hospitals (JCAH) standard on transfer is found in the section on "Emergency Services." The standard states:

> ... no patient should arbitrarily be transferred if the hospital where he was initially seen has means for adequate care of his problem. The patient may not be transferred until the receiving institution has consented to accept the patient. A reasonable record of the immediate medical problem must accompany the patient.[2]

Neither of these statements can be classified as a comprehensive policy on the transfer rights of patients. However, they are a beginning, and hospitals should not hesitate to adopt them as their own policies and adhere to them.

REASONABLE CONDUCT UNDER THE CIRCUMSTANCES

As discussed in Chapter 3 on admission procedures, in deciding whether there is a duty on the part of the hospital and whether that duty has been fulfilled, a court must consider each of the following: (1) the existence of a duty, which may arise by virtue of the hospital's exercise of control over the person, by legislative enactment, or by recognition of an invitation to the public; (2) the nature of the services available at the hospital which would affect the hospital's ability to furnish attention; and (3) a determination of whether the hospital has acted reasonably.

In regard to the transfer of patients, a court would have to focus primarily on the second aspect—that is, the nature of the services available at the hospital which would affect the hospital's ability to furnish attention. The court would, of course, also have to consider the other two issues, duty and reasonable conduct.

How a court looks at the factors is shown in *Jones* v. *City of New York,* 134 N.Y.S. 2d 779 (S. Ct., 1954), modified, 143 N.Y.S. 2d 628 (S. Ct., 1955), in which a woman suffering from a stab wound of the abdomen was taken to the Hospital for Joint Diseases, a charitable hospital. An intern cleaned and dressed the wound and made arrangements to transfer her by ambulance to the City Hospital. She died at City Hospital during an exploratory operation. It was contended that the failure to hospitalize the woman at the first institution and the delay in treatment occasioned by the transfer were contributing causes of death. The court emphasized that her transfer was based on the convenience of City Hospital and not on a determination that her condition was not an emergency. Recovery was permitted against the charitable hospital. The opinion stated:

> . . . the court concludes that the deceased was denied necessary treatment at the Hospital for Joint Diseases and, without her consent, was transferred to the City Hospital and that such transfer was a contributing factor in her death.
> *Jones* v. *City of New York Hospital for Joint Diseases,* 134 N.Y.S.
> 2d 779, 784.

This case seems to indicate that the courts may be more willing to impose a duty on charitable hospitals, and demand a higher standard of care to fulfill that duty, than has been required in the past if one compares it with *O'Neill,* discussed earlier. Both cases also indicate that liability may be imposed when emergency room personnel do not conduct an examination to determine the extent of the injury and thus fail to recognize the severity of the situation.

The applicable standard of care can be ascertained by considering specific cases in which the hospitals have been held liable. Such cases have involved the failure to examine an emergency patient, or to render reasonable care prior to transferring the patient. For example, in a Tennessee case, *Methodist Hospital* v. *Ball,* 50 Tenn. App. 460, 362 S.W. 2d 475 (1961), the court found a hospital negligent when a patient, who had sustained severe injuries in an automobile accident, was left unattended in a corridor for 45 minutes. Then, without an examination, the patient was transferred to another hospital where he died about 15 minutes after arrival. In another case, *New Biloxi Hospital* v. *Frazier,* 245 Miss. 185, 146 So. 2d 882 (1962), the facts show that the patient, bleeding profusely from a gunshot wound, was taken by ambulance to the emergency room. After lengthy delays, he eventually was transferred to the local Veteran's Administration Hospital where he subsequently died. The Mississippi Supreme Court held that a hospital rendering emergency treatment is obliged to do that which is immediately and reasonably necessary to preserve the life and health of the patient, and that it should not discharge a patient in critical condition without furnishing or procuring suitable medical attention.

The Frazier case was based on the negligence of the hospital's nurses and employees in attending and caring for Frazier after he was brought to the hospital's emergency room. Verdict and judgment were for the plaintiff, Frazier's widow, and an appeal was brought. On appeal, the jury's verdict was upheld.

The appellate court outlined the facts in the case. Frazier, a black, was shot in the stump of his left arm, having lost the left arm during World War II. The blast made two large holes in the upper arm and tore away the brachial artery. Bleeding profusely, he was taken by ambulance to the emergency room of the defendant hospital. Ambulance attendants carried him into the emergency room, where one of the nurses just looked at him and walked away. There was blood all over the ambulance cot, and as he waited in the hospital, blood streamed from his arm to the floor, forming a puddle about 24 to 30 inches in diameter. After about 20 minutes another hospital nurse came, looked at Frazier, and walked away.

Shortly after that, at the insistence of the ambulance attendants, the nurses placed Frazier on the table of the emergency room and strapped him down. During all this time, Frazier had been thrashing about and cursing in a nasty manner. The R.N. in charge, Mrs. Perrein, an employee of the hospital, took the patient's blood pressure and pulse. There was no doctor in the hospital on emergency call at the time, so she attempted to call the doctor who was on first emergency call. The first doctor on the list could not be reached; Dr. Smith was contacted and arrived about 30 minutes after being called.

In the meantime, Frazier's wife and several of his friends arrived. They noticed that he was still bleeding and struggling; his wound was unbandaged and there was blood on him and the table. The nurses had made no attempt to stop the bleeding. (Mrs. Perrein later denied Frazier was bleeding, but the jury manifestly found otherwise.) Smith, after looking at the wound and learning that Frazier was a veteran, recommended that he be transferred to the VA Hospital for surgical procedures. Frazier and his wife, although considerably distraught, acquiesced in the transfer. Smith left to obtain an ambulance, but there was considerable delay in getting one.

Neither the nurse nor the doctor made any attempt to stop the bleeding. Dr. Smith testified that he was relying on the nurse to observe the patient and advise him of any changes. He did not take the patient's blood pressure nor did he ask the nurse to do so. He did testify that Frazier had probably started to lapse into shock before he left the hospital.

About two hours after being brought to the emergency room of the defendant hospital, Frazier was transferred by ambulance to the VA hospital. When he arrived, he was practically moribund and, although every type of emergency measure was taken, he was pronounced dead about 30 minutes after arrival. An autopsy revealed that the sole cause of death was hemorrhage with resultant shock. The court stated:

> This summary of the evidence reflects that Frazier was permitted to bleed to death, in the emergency room of appellant's Hospital, through the concurrent negligence of the Hospital's nurses and that of the doctor. The jury was justified in finding that appellant's employees, its nurses, were negligent, and such negligence constituted a proximate contributing cause of Frazier's death in several respects:

> Failure to make any inquiry of the ambulance attendants concerning how long Frazier had been wounded, and how much he had bled; permitting Frazier to bleed unattended on the ambulance cot for an excessive length of time, before even placing him on the emergency room table and examining his wound; failing to take even reasonably simple precautions to diminish or stop the bleeding which was going on, after being placed on the emergency room table; failure of the nurses to advise Dr. Smith, upon his arrival, of the knowledge they had or should have had concerning the amount of bleeding while in the hospital; failing to properly bandage or take other means to stop or reduce the bleeding, after Smith had looked at the wound for a brief time and left the emergency room; and failing to keep a close observation of the patient while waiting for the ambulance to transfer

him to the V.A. Hospital, and to check again his blood pressure and pulse rate.

New Biloxi Hospital, Inc. v. *Frazier,* 146 So. 2d 882 886.

*****

. . . A hospital rendering emergency treatment is obligated to do that which is immediately and reasonably necessary for the preservation of the life, limb or health of the patient. It should not discharge a patient in a critical condition without furnishing or procuring suitable medical attention . . .

New Biloxi Hospital, Inc. v. *Frazier* at page 887.

In the *Jones* case, mentioned earlier, the patient was brought into the emergency room of the defendant hospital suffering from a penetrating wound of the abdomen and minor lacerations of the chest inflicted by an assailant. The intern in charge examined, cleaned, and dressed the wound, and arranged for the patient to be transferred by ambulance to City Hospital. At the receiving hospital she was examined and made ready for exploratory surgery, during the course of which she died, about eight and one-half hours after she had first presented herself for emergency treatment at the defendant hospital. Her estate sued the defendant hospital, alleging that the delay in treatment occasioned by the transfer caused her death, and that the transfer had been made for reasons of hospital convenience, not medical necessity. On appeal, the court found that there was sufficient evidence of the seriousness of the injury and of the defendant hospital's ability to handle such a case. Further, the court found that the decision to transfer was not made for justifiable medical considerations (which would have exonerated the hospital of liability), but rather was made for administrative reasons (which resulted in liability).

The court reached this conclusion after hearing the surgeon at the receiving hospital testify that it would have been more desirable and proper for the patient to have been treated at the defendant hospital, and that her transfer contributed to the condition of shock in which she arrived at City Hospital. The court also heard the testimony of the assistant director of the hospital who said that the ward floors were full, but that there were beds available on private and semiprivate floors, and that the hospital had complete facilities for the surgery required.

In *Methodist Hospital* v. *Ball,* mentioned earlier, the patient was a 16-year-old boy injured while riding in an automobile driven by his mother. He was carried into the emergency room of the Methodist Hospital and remained on a stretcher for approximately 45 minutes while the intern in charge gave instructions to the ambulance driver to take the patient to the emergency room of another hospital. The other hospital was operated primarily as a charity hospital by the City of Memphis. The patient died about 15 minutes after arriving at the second hospital. An autopsy revealed that there was absolutely no evidence of alcohol within his body. Rather the patient had suffered a ruptured liver and internal bleeding as a result of the automobile accident, with a presence of over 3,000 cc of blood in the abdominal cavity.

In its defense, the hospital insisted that it was not liable for the alleged negligent examination and the way the emergency room intern and nurses treated the deceased. The court disagreed, stating that the boy was a patient even though he was never given a room in the hospital and stayed in the emergency room only 45 minutes.

The hospital also argued that it is a physician's privilege to decide between one of two or more courses in the treatment of patients, and a physician cannot be held responsible for an erroneous exercise of judgment. The court agreed with this statement of the law, but added that it must be predicated on the assumption that the physician has exercised ordinary care and skill in examining the patient and in arriving at a diagnosis. The hospital's intern did not meet this test. The court stated:

> . . . we hold there was substantial material evidence upon which the jury might reasonably find Dr. Murphy guilty of negligence: (1) That Dr. Murphy made no examination of young Ball but simply accepted the opinion of one or more persons in the emergency room that young Ball was only drunk and not injured, or (2) that Dr. Murphy did examine Ball, diagnosed his condition as critical and having possible internal injuries and yet gave him no supportive treatment of any kind, failed to make any attempt to alert the personnel at John Gaston Hospital of his critical condition . . .
> *Methodist Hospital* v. *Ball,* 362 S.W. 2d 475, 487.

In *Hunt* v. *Palm Springs General Hospital,* 352 So. 2d 582 (Fla. Dist. Ct. App., 1977), a state appeals court addressed the issue of whether a private hospital owed a duty of care to a patient it did not officially admit, but who died following transfer by the hospital to another facility. Admission had been refused since the patient was in debt to the hospital for care previously rendered and was not believed to be critically ill. Noting that the patient lay trembling in the hospital hallway for several hours with an elevated blood pressure and pulse rate, the court ruled that a jury should determine whether the hospital had a duty to render medical care, and whether there had been any breach of such duty which was a causative factor in Hunt's death.

A review of these cases emphasizes that in transferring patients, as in situations of admission and discharge, hospitals should not make the transfer when doing so would risk the person's life or safety. Clearly then, transfers for the convenience of the hospital are very risky. Also, where it is foreseeable that a person requires emergency treatment and a transfer would cause a delay in treatment, the transfer should not occur.

This issue of foreseeability was important in a recent Florida case. In *Nance v. James Archer Smith Hospital, Inc.,* 329 So. 2d 377 (Fla. App., 1976), a wrongful death action was brought against the defendant hospital. The facts in this unfortunate case show that a young male was behaving strangely at home. His grandmother became concerned and, with two of the young man's friends, took her grandson to the emergency department of the defendant hospital. It appeared that the grandson had taken a pill containing LSD. The hospital personnel were informed that the boy had taken "acid." The ward clerk advised the grandmother that the hospital did not have the proper testing facilities to ascertain the type of drug her grandson had taken, and thus she should take him to another hospital that did have the necessary testing facilities. Thereupon, the grandmother and companions began to drive the grandson to the second hospital. Shortly thereafter, the grandson jumped out of the car, ran berserk through an apartment building, and fatally stabbed Ernest Nance.

Margaret Nance, wife of the victim, filed a wrongful death action against the hospital, alleging that the hospital was negligent in turning the boy away inasmuch as he was a danger to himself and others. Although the jury returned a verdict of $150,000 in favor of Mrs. Nance, the trial judge, having reserved ruling of the defendant hospital's motion for a directed verdict, entered judgment for the hospital. The court stated:

> The record is replete with evidence that Franklin, during the time he was present at the defendant hospital, did not exhibit any behavior which could be termed erratic or threatening and we conclude there was no reasonable foreseeability that Franklin would engage in the violent behavior which resulted in the death of plaintiff's husband.
> *Nance v. James Archer Smith Hospital, Inc.,* 329 So. 2d
> 377 (Fla. App., 1976)

This case is interesting because it shows the importance the court placed on the boy's conduct while in the defendant hospital. It seems clear that had there been evidence of erratic behavior while in the hospital, the outcome could very well have been different, with the court holding the hospital liable, which the jury was certainly willing to do.

ABANDONMENT

The charge of abandonment can arise during the transfer of a patient from the emergency department of one hospital to the emergency department of a second hospital. To minimize its exposure to charges of negligence and abandonment, the transferring hospital must assume the responsibility of stabilizing the patient's condition, examining the patient to determine whether the patient can tolerate transferral, arranging for the receiving hospital to approve the transfer, arranging with the patient to approve the transfer, and giving the patient supportive treatment until she or he is accepted as a patient by the receiving hospital.

Emergency departments should clearly outline in their policies and procedures the protocol to be followed when patients are transferred. These policies should address four issues: (1) the reasons for transfer, including when transfer is recommended by the hospital and when it is requested by the patient; (2) the need for an initial examination to determine the patient's condition and the need for transferral; (3) any statutory requirements on transferral; and (4) the need for interhospital agreements on patient transfers, including the need for a transfer summary that summarizes the patient's status, reason for transfer, and any other pertinent information a receiving hospital should have.

NOTES

1. Mary Cazalas, *Nursing and the Law,* 3rd ed. (Germantown, Md.: Aspen Systems Corporation, 1978), p. 142.

2. Joint Commission on Accreditation of Hospitals, *Accreditation Manual for Hospitals,* February 1978 ed., (Chicago: JCAH, 1978), p. 15.

PART III

Death and Discharge

Chapter 6

Death in the Emergency Room

Although patient deaths occur in all departments of a general hospital, on the general wards there is often time to prepare the patient, family and friends, and the staff. In contrast, in the emergency department death is usually the result of a sudden outside force that is not expected and therefore overwhelming.

This chapter will deal with the many issues involved in the death of emergency room patients. Issues such as reporting requirements, notification of next of kin, disposal of the body, and autopsy requirements will be discussed in detail.

By its very nature, emergency care is short-term. Patients are treated immediately for whatever symptoms are life-threatening; if they need continuing care, they are transferred to other appropriate departments of the hospital. If death occurs, it is usually within a relatively short period of time. Therefore, whether the outcome of a patient visit is survival or death, the staff has relatively brief, albeit intense, contact with the patient.

Generally, the issues involving death of emergency patients, the right to possession of the deceased patient, and control of the body for purposes of burial are controlled by state law. Thus laws will vary from state to state. The policies of an emergency department on such matters as death of patients, including those dead on arrival, should be in accordance with state laws. In order to assure this, the hospital should seek the advice of local counsel before such policies are drafted and put into effect.

In most states, laws require only that the attending physician complete a death certificate when the patient dies. The next of kin should, of course, be notified immediately or as soon as is reasonably possible. The duty to inform patients extends to the next of kin.

An autopsy should not be performed until the nearest relative grants permission *in writing*. Permission for autopsy can also be obtained from appropriate officials as designated by state laws. Legal authority to perform an autopsy bars objections from relatives.

EMOTIONAL ISSUES

The death of a patient always involves emotional issues. In the emergency room the nature of care requires that the staff focus on the physical needs of patients in order to save their lives. In a true emergency, these physical needs are so urgent there is little time to think about patients' emotional needs.

In situations where emergency patients are disoriented but conscious, it is important to orient them by explaining in a calm, reassuring manner that they are in an emergency room and why they are there. Some patients brought to an emergency department in critical condition may be unconscious or in shock; they may be unaware of what is happening to them and around them. In these situations there may be little if any patient-staff interaction.

Other patients admitted in critical condition may be very well oriented, may know exactly where they are and why, and may be concerned about the prognosis. Clearly, these patients need reassurance. However, more than reassurance, they need to know they will not be left alone. In emergency departments with an ombudsman, it can be the ombudsman's responsibility to stay with the patient. Dying patients fear dying alone. Emergency staff members should be alert to this fear and should make certain that dying patients are not left unattended.

Commentators and writers on death and dying seem to be in agreement that dying patients should never be told they are dying. This creates tension for staff members because a dying patient will often ask if he or she is dying. The staff member may be faced with a real dilemma. Although there is no easy answer to this problem, emergency room physicians and nurses will find that the best way to answer this kind of question is to assess the patient's needs. Some patients who ask this question really may not want a truthful answer; some, of course, do. There is no blanket policy right for every patient. Staff members should, however, try to assure patients that everything possible is being done to prevent death and that they will not be left alone.

While life-saving measures are being taken and after death has occurred, the family and friends should not be forgotten. Emergency staff members can be so focused on the patient that the family is temporarily ignored. However, when a patient has expired, the family must be told. In emergency rooms, where deaths are often sudden, families often have not had adequate time to prepare for the death of a loved one. They need more, not less, staff time than families of patients who take days, weeks, or months to die.

Some emergency departments have arranged for social workers to be available to give support to the family and friends of a deceased patient. But given the costs involved and the fact that many of these situations occur at odd hours (on holidays, weekends, and other times when social workers are not on duty), this is more the exception than the rule.

When death occurs in the emergency room, there is a real need to provide a private area for the grieving family. Many emergency departments do not provide a private area because of limited space. Each emergency department needs to assess its own case load to determine how often such an area is needed. Surely, emergency departments that see a reasonably large number of deaths, including patients dead on arrival, should arrange for some space for grieving relatives. If space is not available in the emergency department itself, perhaps unused office space or a chapel could be used.

What happens when the family is not with the dying or deceased patient? Many commentators feel that it is bad policy to notify a family by phone that a relative has died unexpectedly. The family may react hysterically or irrationally as a result. Commentators feel that it is better to call calmly with news of the accident and ask the family to come to the hospital without telling them of the death.

Another alternative might be to telephone the family and inform them of the accident and the death in the most sympathetic way possible. The caller should stress that everything possible was done for the deceased, and that there is nothing to be accomplished by the family coming to the hospital. If the family insists on coming to the hospital, the caller should urge them to take a cab or have a friend drive them; under no circumstances should they drive themselves because of the very real possibility that their emotional distress may cause them to have an accident while traveling. The caller can suggest they contact a friend or another relative to be with them.

A funeral director chosen by the family can pick up the body and bring it wherever the family wishes. If there is a problem with identification of the body, the caller can suggest that a friend of the family or a minister come to identify the deceased—someone who is not as closely connected with the decedent in an emotional way, but who could make the identification. The hospital should have facilities to keep the body for a reasonable length of time until arrangements can be made for a funeral, etc.

DEAD ON ARRIVAL CASES

Patients brought to a hospital emergency department dead on arrival (DOA) must be reported to the coroner or medical examiner of the locality or political subdivision in which the death occurred.

Because such cases come under the jurisdiction of the coroner or medical examiner, the body, clothing, and any other belongings must be turned over to the coroner's office. It is important to not alter the corpse in any way prior to notification of the coroner. It is the responsibility of the coroner or medical examiner to conduct an investigation to determine the possibility of foul play and whether an autopsy or post-mortem investigation is advised.

In these cases it is the responsibility of the emergency room physician to pronounce death of the patient. If there is any question of life, all attempts should be made to preserve life, including resuscitative measures.

The medical record should include all known information about the cause of death plus any signs of trauma or injury. If the deceased is unidentified, emergency room physicians should label the record as Jane or John Doe until identification is made.

In DOA cases, although pronouncement of death may be made by the emergency room physician, the death certificate must be signed by the medical examiner. When a medical examiner or coroner takes responsibility for the case, by law his or her authority overrides that of the emergency room physician, attending physician, spouse, or other next of kin.

MEDICAL EXAMINER'S OR CORONER'S CASES

State laws govern when a death comes under the jurisdiction of the medical examiner or coroner. Generally, the following cases are reportable to the office of coroner or medical examiner. The office will determine whether or not to assume jurisdiction.

- All suicides
- All DOAs
- All violent deaths
- All deaths without prior medical care
- All deaths resulting from poisoning
- All deaths resulting from criminal acts
- All deaths wherein patients have been hospitalized for less than 24 hours and a definite diagnosis has not been made
- All deaths for which an attending physician cannot or will not sign the death certificate

- All deaths resulting from an accident
- All deaths wherein the patient has not been seen by the attending physician for 20 days or more prior to death

The state laws are fairly uniform from state to state. Emergency personnel should familiarize themselves with the exact requirements for their state and, when in doubt, consult local counsel.

When the medical examiner or coroner assumes jurisdiction of a death, the signing of the death certificate and the authorization for and extent of an autopsy become solely the responsibility of the coroner or medical examiner. He or she may, by law, delegate the signing of the death certificate or the performance of the autopsy, but the coroner or medical examiner retains complete responsibility.

It is important for emergency departments to be in compliance with the law in this area. To assure this, department policies and procedures should address the issue of DOAs and other deaths reportable to the medical examiner or coroner.

DEATH IN GENERAL

It is unlikely that problems caused by the use of maintenance medical systems can be resolved until a precise definition of death is found—a definition that is acceptable to both the legal and medical professions. In 1975 the American Bar Association, in an attempt toward clarification, adopted the following resolution: "... for all legal purposes, a human body with irreversible cessation of total brain function, according to usual and customary standards of medical practice, shall be considered dead."

However, the American Medical Association has refused to adopt a definition of death and continues to maintain that the individual physician should decide when death has occurred by relying on sound medical custom. In the not too distant past, this meant the absence of a heartbeat and the cessation of respiration. But medical procedures have been developing at breakneck speed, and the currently recognized (albeit unsanctioned) definition seems to be brain death, by which is meant the irreversible cessation of brain function. The criteria generally used to determine this condition have been those established in 1968 by the Ad Hoc Committee of the Harvard Medical School to Examine the Definition of Brain Death. This committee's report lists four characteristics of irreversible coma that, if verified, would constitute brain death:

1. Unreceptivity and unresponsivity. The patient fails to respond to any external stimuli regardless of the painful nature of the stimuli.
2. No movement or breathing. After observation by physicians for at least one hour the patient does not move or breathe spontaneously or respond in any way to pain, touch, sound or light. To establish the non-spontaneous breathing of a person being maintained by a respirator, the machine may be turned off for a test period of three minutes.
3. No reflexes. The patient's pupils are fixed, dilated and unresponsive to direct light while occular movement fails to respond to ice water irrigation of the ear canal. Swallowing, blinking, yawning and vocalization are absent. No tendon reflexes can be elicited.
4. Flat electroencephalogram (EEG). It is suggested that the EEG be utilized for its confirmatory value. The test should be run for at least ten minutes; however, twice that time is considered preferable and the test should be repeated at least 24 hours later with no changes appearing. There should be no electroencephalogram response to noise or to a pinch. The test results will be invalid if the patient has ingested central nervous system depressants such as barbiturates or has experienced hypothermia (temperature below 90 degrees F or 32.2 degrees C).[1]

The Supreme Judicial Court of Massachusetts, in *Commonwealth* v. *Golston,* 366 N.E. 2d 744, cert. denied, 434 U.S. 1039 (1977), recognized the Harvard Ad Hoc Committee's definition of "brain death." The three basic clinical criteria for meeting this definition, the court stated, are unresponsiveness to normally painful stimuli, absence of spontaneous movements or breathing, and absence of reflexes—all confirmed by an electroencephalogram and observation over a 24-hour period. Although the court accepted the "brain death" definition in this case, the court emphasized that "brain death" was a factor only as it affected conviction, this being a criminal case. In a later case, however, the same court cited *Golston,* noting that the brain death criteria had been "recently recognized by this court as a medically and legally acceptable definition of death."

Because of the importance in defining death for purposes of medical treatment, organ transplants, and the movement toward right-to-die legislation, there is a clear trend for state legislatures to redefine death by statute. New statutes are replacing the traditional definition of cessation of circulation and respiration with a definition of cessation of brain activity. For example, the recently enacted New Mexico statute, N.M. Stat. Ann, Sec. 1-2-2.2 (Supp. 1973; S.B. No. 16 (Laws 1977) reads as follows:

Sec. 1-2-2.2 Death Defined.

For all medical, legal and statutory purposes death of a human being occurs when, and "death," "dead body," "dead person," or any other reference to human death means that:

(1) based on ordinary standards of medical practice, there is the absence of spontaneous respiratory and cardiac function and, because of the disease or condition which caused, directly or indirectly, these functions to cease, or because of the passage of time since these functions ceased, there is not reasonable possibility of restoring respiratory or cardiac functions; in this event death occurs at the time respiratory or cardiac functions ceased; or

(2) in the opinion of a physician, based on ordinary standards of medical practice; (a) because of a known disease or condition there is absence of spontaneous brain function; and (b) after reasonable attempt to either maintain or restore spontaneous circulatory or respiratory functions in the absence of spontaneous brain function, it appears that further attempts at resuscitation and supportive maintenance have no reasonable possibility of restoring spontaneous brain function; in this event death will have occurred at the time when the absence of spontaneous brain function first occurred. Death is to be pronounced pursuant to this paragraph before artificial means of supporting respiratory or circulatory functions are terminated and before any vital organ is removed for purposes of transplantation in compliance with the Uniform Anatomical Gift Act (12-11-6 to 12-11-14).

B. The alternative definitions of death in paragraphs (1) and (2) of subsection A of this section are to be utilized for all purposes in this state, including but not limited to civil and criminal actions, notwithstanding any other law to the contrary.

At the present time, only a minority of states have defined death in terms of irreversible cessation of brain function, as has New Mexico. But it is a definite trend, and we can expect more and more states to do the same.

At the same time that state legislatures are grappling with definitions, state courts are defining death when presented with the question. Two recent cases show that brain death is evolving as the legal definition of death.

In a highly publicized Oregon murder case, *State* v. *Brown,* 8 Oreg. App. 72, 491 P. 2d 1193 (1971), the defendant argued that death was not caused by a bullet wound inflicted by the defendant, but by the physician who removed the mechanisms artificially supporting the victim's circulation and respiration.

The court rejected defendant's argument and held that death was caused by brain wound as a result of the bullet and not by the removal of life-support systems.

One year later, in a Virginia case, a jury was allowed to choose between two definitions in determining the actual time of death. One was the traditional definition; the other was the brain death definition. The jury chose the latter.

Clearly, this is a dynamic area, and the law is not yet settled. For emergency room personnel, determination of the time of death is an important area insofar as organ transplants are involved.

DONATIONS OF BODIES

The Commissioners on Uniform State Laws, in recognition of the possible liability for physicians and organizations that obtain and use bodies and body parts for medical purposes, including transplantation, drafted a Uniform Anatomical Gift Act that has been endorsed by the American Bar Association. Many states have subsequently enacted this act as state law. The law details many provisions for the making, acceptance, and use of anatomical gifts.

The donation laws usually permit donors to execute the gift during their lifetimes and preclude liability on the part of surviving relatives for use of the body in conformity with the donation. In order to be effective legally, the donor must abide by the statutory requirements. These laws generally have two purposes. One is to effectuate the wishes of the deceased, and the other is to provide liability immunity to the donee of the gift. A donee, acting pursuant to a gift that is not valid because it does not comply with the statutory requirements, would appear to be subject to liability to the surviving relatives for interference with their interests in the body of the deceased. Thus some state statutes provide that where a gift does not comply with the statutory requirements, the wishes of the decedent should nevertheless be honored.

In some of the states that have not enacted the Uniform Anatomical Gift Act, there are statutes that specifically authorize donations of bodies or body parts by the deceased prior to death. Some state laws are limited only to the donation of eyes.

In states lacking a Uniform Anatomical Gift Act, the wishes of the surviving relatives may be in conflict with the wishes of the deceased. It is recognized that surviving relatives do have an interest in the body of the deceased patient. In these situations, it is best to obtain written permission from the surviving relatives.

The Uniform Anatomical Gift Act provides that the physician who declares the patient dead cannot be a member of the transplant team. This requirement addresses the possible conflict of interest on the part of physicians. It is designed to ensure that the interests of the possible donor will be fully protected by physicians with responsibility for his welfare and not that of the possible recipient.

It is necessary to remove body organs and tissues almost immediately after death. Recommended removal time for eyes for corneal transplant is within one hour of death. Therefore, it is imperative that agreement or arrangement for obtaining organs and tissue from a body be completed before death or immediately after death.

Very often, in emergency departments, because of various factors, the staff does not know of or learn of the intended anatomical gift. This is a special hazard in hospital emergency departments located in metropolitan areas near heavily traveled highways. Because of sudden, unexpected deaths as a result of accidents, because of our highly mobile society, and because of the very nature of emergency care—which is not extended care as with a trusted family physician—there are times when gifts are not made because no one knows of the deceased's wishes. Often, by the time someone does find identification or other information, it is too late to remove the body parts. Some states are attempting to alleviate this problem by placing information concerning donation on the person's driver's license.

Donors

Under the Uniform Anatomical Gift Act, a donor must be at least 18 years of age and of sound mind. The gift or donation may be made by will or other written instrument and may specify the body parts donated. The act allows donation for purposes of education, therapy, transplantation, or for the advancement of medical or dental science.

The act provides for donation by the next of kin, in a statutory preference order, if consent has not been obtained from the decedent prior to death. If consent is obtained after death from relatives, the statute provides for consent by recorded message. The statute provides that when only a part of the body is donated, custody of the remaining parts of the body is to be transferred to the next of kin promptly following removal of the donated part.

Donees

Hospitals, surgeons, medical and dental schools, colleges and universities, tissue banks or storage facilities, or specified individuals for needed therapy or transplantation are specifically made eligible donees by the Uniform Anatomical Gift Act.

Revocation

The statute provides several methods by which the donation may be revoked. If the document has been delivered to a named donee, it may be revoked by (1) a written revocation signed by the donor and delivered to the donee; (2) an oral revocation witnessed by two persons and communicated to the donee; (3) a statement made to the attending physician and communicated to the donee during a terminal illness or (4) a card or written statement signed by the donor and carried on his or her person or in his or her immediate effects. If the written instrument of donation has not been delivered to the donee, it may be revoked by destruction, cancellation, or mutilation of the instrument. If the donation is made by a will, it may be revoked in the manner provided for revocation of wills. Any person acting in good faith reliance on the terms of an instrument of donation will not be subject to civil or criminal liability unless that person has actual notice of the revocation.

POSSESSION OF THE BODY

The rule now uniformly recognized in this country is that the person entitled to possession of a body for the purpose of burial has certain legally protected interests. The development of these rights has been summarized in 22 Am. Jur. 2d Dead Bodies § 4 (1965), as follows:

> . . . In fact the early common law of England recognized no property or property rights in the body of a deceased person, this being due, undoubtedly, to the fact that the ecclesiastical courts exercized jurisdiction over the affairs of decedents. Although this doctrine has found some support in early American cases, the established rule is that notwithstanding there can be no property right in a dead body in the commercial sense, there is a quasi-property right in dead bodies vesting in the nearest relatives of the deceased and arising out of their duty to bury their dead. This right, which corresponds in extent to the duty out of which it arises, includes the right to possession and custody of the body for burial, the right to have it remain in its final resting place so the memory of the deceased may receive the respect of the living, or to remove the body to a proper place, and the right to maintain an action to recover damages for any outrage, indignity or injury to the body of the deceased.

Damages awarded in cases where liability is predicated on interference with the rights of a surviving spouse or near relative in the body of a decedent are based on emotional and mental suffering that results from such interference. Thus, for damages to be awarded in these cases, the conduct of the alleged wrongdoer must be sufficiently disturbing to cause emotional harm to a person of ordinary sensibilities.

In *Muniz* v. *United Hospitals Medical Center—Presbyterian Hospital,* 153 N.J. Super. 79, 379 A. 2d 57 (1977), a New Jersey appeals court overturned a trial court decision, and held that the parents of a premature infant born at one hospital but who died at another hospital after transfer there for special treatment may sue the second hospital for emotional distress stemming from inappropriate handling of the infant's body and from the hospital's method of informing them of the baby's death. After notifying the mother by phone of her two-day-old infant's death, the hospital allegedly failed to confirm the death or locate the body for a period of three weeks. The court took exception to the trial court's refusal to expand New Jersey's law of negligence, which only permits recovery for emotional distress that is occasioned by a reasonable fear of immediate personal injury. It reasoned that the parents may have a claim for emotional distress that is based on one of several possible grounds, including: a property right to the child's corpse; an implied contract with the hospital; the tort of outrage; or a breach of the hospital's standard of care in dealing with corpses, such that emotional distress would be a foreseeable consequence.

Refusal to deliver a dead body to a proper person who demands custody of the body has also resulted in liability. While there do not appear to be any such cases directly involving hospitals, if a hospital refused to deliver a body until the decedent's bill was paid, or retained possession of a body after a proper request for delivery, such refusal would constitute sufficient grounds upon which to sue for liability for interference with rights to a dead body. In *Gratton* v. *Baldwinsville Academy and Central School,* 49 Misc. 2d 329, 267 N.Y.S. 2d 552 (1966), the school's refusal for some three or four minutes to permit a mother to view the body of her dead child because the body was being held for the coroner was held to be an actionable wrong. The court stated that the law is well settled that the surviving next of kin have a right to the immediate possession of a decedent's body for preservation and burial. This New York case emphasizes the fact that hospital policies and procedures in handling dead bodies must be consistent with the interests of the deceased's relatives.

Although several persons may suffer emotional stress and mental suffering because of indignities stemming from improper handling of the body of the decedent, recovery for wrongful interference with the body and proper burial of the body has generally been limited to the person who has the right to possession of the body for burial. In some states there are statutes that delineate an order for devolution of the duty to bury the decedent. Other states have provisions setting forth an order of persons authorized to give consent to autopsy, from which the order of devolution may be established. In states without either type of provision, case law must provide the guidelines. Generally the primary right to custody of a dead body belongs to the surviving spouse. When there is no spouse, the right devolves upon the children of the decedent, if any, and then upon the decedent's parents.

It should be recognized that hospitals may be held liable for improper handling of dead bodies by mislabeling or confusing identification and tagging of bodies. This involves unintentional as well as intentional conduct. In *Lott v. State,* 32 Misc. 2d 296, 225 N.Y.S. 2d 434 (1962), a hospital was held liable for mental anguish that resulted from negligent conduct that interfered with burial plans. The negligent conduct consisted of mistagging two bodies, which resulted in the preparation of a person of the Roman Catholic faith for an Orthodox Jewish burial and a person of the Orthodox Jewish faith for a Roman Catholic burial. Each decedent's family was awarded $1,000 for the emotional upset caused by such matters as the embalming and use of cosmetics in violation of religious beliefs, having to return the body to the hospital mortuary and having to examine other bodies, having to identify their mother's body, and having to make new arrangements for the funeral.

UNCLAIMED DEAD BODIES

Persons entitled to possession of a dead body must arrange for release of the body from the hospital, for its transfer to an embalmer or undertaker, and for its final disposal. The recognition by the courts of a quasi-property right in the body of a deceased person imposes a duty on the hospital to make reasonable efforts to give notice to persons entitled to claim the body. When there are no known relatives or friends of the family who can be contacted by the hospital to claim the body, the hospital has the responsibility to dispose of the body in accordance with law.

Unclaimed bodies are generally buried at public expense. A public official, usually a county official, has the duty to bury or otherwise dispose of such bodies. Most states have statutes providing for the disposal of unclaimed bodies by delivery to institutions for educational and scientific purposes. Thus, unclaimed bodies in the custody of public officials, such as coroners or administrators of governmental hospitals, are subject to use for such purposes. Pursuant to these statutes, the public official in charge of the body has a duty to notify the government agency of the presence of the body. The agency then arranges for the transfer of the body in accordance with the statute. If no such agency exists under the statute, the hospital or public official may be authorized to allow a medical school or other institution or person designated by the statute as an eligible recipient of unclaimed dead bodies to remove the body for scientific use.

When an unclaimed dead body is in the possession of a charitable or proprietary hospital, the hospital should notify the public official charged by law with the duty to dispose of unclaimed bodies. The public official then arranges for the ultimate disposition of the body, either by burial or by transfer to an institution entitled to obtain it for educational and scientific purposes.

Certain categories of persons are usually excluded from the provisions that permit the distribution of bodies for educational and scientific use. For public health reasons, the statutes usually prohibit distribution of the bodies of persons who died from contagious diseases. Generally, the bodies of travelers and veterans also are not to be used for educational and scientific purposes.

While the majority of these statutes state quite explicitly the requirements for notifying relatives and the time limits for holding the body to allow relatives an opportunity to claim it, strict compliance with the statutory provisions is often impossible due to the required procedures themselves and to the very nature of the problems that arise in handling dead bodies. Noncompliance in such instances would not appear to cause liability. An example of such a provision is the requirement that relatives be notified immediately upon death and that the body be held for 24 hours subject to claim by a relative or friend. The procedure of locating and notifying relatives may consume the greater part of the 24-hour period following death, and if relatives who are willing to claim the body are located, the body should be held for a reasonable time to allow them to obtain custody of the body for burial. The hospital should recognize that literal compliance may prejudice the interests of relatives of the decedent.

Similarly, where a body remains unclaimed and the hospital has no way of ascertaining that the decedent was a veteran, delivering or disposing of the body for educational or scientific purposes pursuant to the statute would not appear to cause liability should it later be proved the decedent was a veteran.

In some instances the hospital may be or may desire to become a recipient of cadaveric material to be used for scientific or educational purposes. This may be true in respect to bodies of persons held by public officials and other hospitals, as well as the unclaimed bodies of persons who died within the recipient institution. In either case, should a hospital desire such materials, it must comply with the statutory provisions relating to recipients. Such provisions may require that the hospital register as an eligible recipient or request that a bond be given to insure proper use and disposal of the body. In addition, to qualify as a recipient the hospital may be required to maintain equipment and facilities for the preservation and storage of cadavers.

It can be seen that emergency department policies and procedures must address both the issues of death in the emergency room and coroner or medical examiner cases. These policies and procedures need to cover at least the following:

- reportable deaths

- disposal of bodies

- morgue procedures

- coroner or medical examiner procedures

- police procedures

- next of kin notification procedures

- donation of body and body parts procedures

- identification of the body procedures

- medical record and release form procedures

- autopsy procedures

AUTOPSY

The purpose of conducting an autopsy is to determine the cause of a person's death. The autopsy or post-mortem examination is thus able to determine many legal issues: whether death resulted from criminal acts; whether the cause of death was one for which payment is due under an insurance contract; whether the cause of death is compensable under workmen's compensation and occupational disease acts; or whether death resulted from one specific act or a culmination of several acts. There is a second justification for the performance of autopsies or post-mortem examinations. Autopsies are necessary to hospitals, physicians and nurses, and medical science because they offer a tremendous learning opportunity. Furthermore, the results of autopsies are often used as a check on the medical practice in the hospital. The Joint Commission on Accreditation of Hospitals desires that autopsies be performed on the bodies of at least 20 percent of the persons dying within each hospital, and the American Medical Association requires an autopsy rate of at least 25 percent in facilities and institutions approved for intern training.

Any type of autopsy, whether or not it includes tissue removal, requires consent. It is a long accepted principle that consent obtained through fraud or material misrepresentation is not legally binding, and that the person whose consent is so obtained stands in the same position as if no consent had been given.

Sometimes the facts are misrepresented to the person possessing the right to consent in order to induce his or her consent. Where a physician or hospital employee states as fact something known to be untrue in order to gain consent, the autopsy would be unauthorized and liability may follow. A statement that hospital rules require an autopsy when this is not so would constitute a misrepresentation of fact that could invalidate the consent.

In *Grawunder* v. *Beth Israel Hospital Ass'n.*, 266 N.Y. 605, 195 N.E. 221 (1935), the hospital defended an action for an unauthorized autopsy by introducing into evidence its rules stating that autopsies were not to be performed without consent, testimony of its pathologist and his assistants that neither he nor they performed an autopsy on the deceased, and testimony of its medical director to the effect that no member of the staff performed the autopsy and that the body of the deceased was in the hospital's morgue, the key to which was in the hospital's office. The court affirmed a verdict for the plaintiff, holding that though a hospital is not an insurer of the safety of a corpse, the evidence clearly showed that the body, which was in the possession of the hospital from the time of death until it was picked up by the undertaker, was mutilated while in the exclusive possession and control of the hospital. Thus the hospital, though it had no knowledge of the unauthorized autopsy, was held responsible because it enjoyed exclusive control of the body and had the means to know what might have been done to it.

However, in *Hasselback* v. *Mount Sinai Hospital*, 173 App. Div. 89, 159 N.Y. Supp. 376 (1916), with facts somewhat similar to those of the *Grawunder* case, judgment for the hospital was affirmed because the plaintiff, in her demurrer, admitted that the unauthorized autopsy was not performed by an agent of the hospital. Therefore, the court reasoned the question to be decided was only whether or not the hospital owed an absolute duty to the plaintiff to protect her husband's body from mutilation. The court refused to impose an absolute duty on the hospital.

Both these cases emphasize that a hospital must take precautions to prevent unauthorized autopsy and other wrongful use of a body. It should also be noted that the *Hasselback* case (in which the hospital was found not liable) was decided 19 years before the *Grawunder* case (in which the hospital was found liable). Thus the later case is the better authority. In general, recovery for emotional trauma has been permitted more often in later years.

While most cases concerning unauthorized autopsies have been brought against persons actually performing the autopsy, and the statutes that deal with autopsies and rights to custody of dead bodies do not specifically direct hospitals to obtain consent, such cases and statutes should be consulted in determining prudent hospital procedures with respect to autopsies.

Autopsy Consent Statutes

Most states have enacted statutes dealing with autopsy consent. This legislation has two intentions: (1) to afford protection to the rights of the decedent's relatives; and (2) to serve as a guide for hospitals and physicians in establishing procedures for consent to autopsy.

Autopsy consent statutes vary from state to state, and so it is important for emergency department personnel to be cognizant of the requirements in the state in which they practice their professions. There is no uniformity among state statutes in states that have enacted them; there are also some states that have not enacted legislation in this area. In general, the usual priority for consent is as follows: the surviving spouse; surviving children over the age of 18 years; the surviving parents of the deceased; the surviving siblings of majority age of the deceased; other surviving adult relatives in order of closest blood relationship.

If the death is a coroner's or medical examiner's case, the request for the autopsy must be signed by an official of the coroner's or medical examiner's office. (See Exhibit 6-1 for a sample autopsy authorization form.) A request signed by any other person is ineffective. The autopsy permit must be signed and witnessed and should specify any limitations or restrictions. Any such limitations or restrictions must be adhered to by the pathologist who performs the autopsy.

Approximately half of the autopsy consent statutes provide that the deceased may authorize an autopsy on his or her own body. Such consent should be in writing. Because of the sudden and unexpected nature of deaths that occur in emergency departments, this matter should rarely, if ever, arise.

In states where there is neither an autopsy consent statute nor a statute permitting donation that may be construed to include autopsy, it is unwise to rely solely on the authorization of a decedent to perform an autopsy. This is especially true where there is an objection to autopsy on the part of the relatives of the deceased who assume custody of the body for burial. Although many cases have upheld the decedent's wishes with respect to the place of interment or the manner of disposition of the remains (that is, burial or cremation), the courts may not afford the same weight to a deceased's wishes concerning autopsy. In such instances, compelling reasons presented by certain kin of the decedent, and especially the surviving spouse, may prevail over the wishes of the decedent. For these reasons, the hospital should always attempt to secure authorization from the decedent's relatives or any other person who assumes custody of the body, even if authorization has been given by the decedent, unless there is a statute that specifically declares that a decedent's authorization is sufficient in itself.

Exhibit 6-1 Sample Autopsy Authorization Form

Authorization for Autopsy*

_____ Date_____19____p.m.
Name of deceased   a.m.

I, _____, as nearest of kin to the deceased, hereby
authorize the _____ Hospital of _____
                                              city
____, _____, its employees, agents, and representatives,
        state
to conduct a post-mortem examination upon the body of the
deceased, including the removal and retention of such organs and
parts of such organs and tissues as may be deemed proper by the
examining physician in the interests of determining the cause of
death and of advancing medical knowledge and progress.

Witnesses

_____   _____
                                        signature

_____   _____
                                        relationship

* If it is known that the arrangements for burial are being made by
a person other than the next of kin, obtain an additional Authorization
for Autopsy from that person. Strike out the words "nearest of" if
such person is a relative. Strike out the phrase "as nearest of kin to
the deceased" if such person is not related.

Occasions arise in which the first person in order of preference is deceased, mentally incompetent, unwilling, unable, or fails to assume responsibility for burial of the body. It is then necessary to descend the preference order to determine who has such responsibility and the concomitant right to authorize the performance of an autopsy. Fortunately, in many states the order of responsibility for burial is set forth in statutes, and the right to authorize the hospital to perform an autopsy is given to the person who has assumed custody of the body for burial. Several statutes that specifically deal with authority for autopsies indicate who should be sought out to give authorization should the first person in order of priority be unavailable. Such statutes enable the hospital to determine whose consent is sufficient. If the statutory provisions are followed, the chance of a successful suit by one claiming superior rights is practically nonexistent.

Where the person who is highest on the preference order assumes custody of the body for burial and refuses to authorize an autopsy, the consent of other persons lower on the preference order is ineffective. Such persons do not have rights to the body under such circumstances. Valid consent to autopsy can only be given by the person who has the authority to give consent.

It is important to note that in a typical emergency department situation, requesting an autopsy can be a situation fraught with strain due to the fact that the relatives of the deceased were not prepared for the death. In addition, the request for an autopsy may be made by a physician who is a virtual stranger, as contrasted to a family physician well known to the family. In these situations, the person requesting consent for an autopsy must take extra precautions to be most sensitive, calm, and understanding in explaining why an autopsy is needed and advised.

NOTE

1. Ad Hoc Committee of Harvard Law School, "Autopsy and Donation," in *Hospital Law Manual* (Germantown, Md.: November 1977), p. 2(4).

Chapter 7

Discharge Policies
and Procedures

It has been claimed, justifiably, that the two major problems that arise with respect to discharging persons from hospitals relate to the exercise of restraint on patients who desire to leave and the discharge of patients whose health or safety may be endangered by leaving the hospital.

These two problems may be more acute in an emergency department than in any other department of a general hospital. This is due to the nature of emergency health care. Emergency department staff members see patients—often unknown to them—over a short period of time, for sudden and unexpected illnesses and accidents. In the midst of seeing a large volume of patients, it is possible that patients will be discharged prematurely, or less frequently, retained longer than necessary.

If, after some treatment has been rendered, a hospital emergency department removes a person from the premises, it may be considered a failure to admit the person for full hospital services rather than an improper discharge. Cases of this nature have been treated as admission cases in Chapter 3 where the facts clearly indicated that the sick or injured person remained in the hospital emergency department for a very short period of time. Cases involving a longer stay or issues of proper discharge are considered in this chapter in terms of the propriety of the discharge. Whether viewed as in improper discharge or an admission failure, the critical issue is whether the hospital's conduct created an unreasonable risk of harm.

It is important to understand this issue. If it were not that unwarranted discharge could risk a patient's health and safety, there would not be a problem as to when to discharge. However, discharging a person who is obviously still in need of care or treatment or who clearly is incompetent of self-care does risk the person's health and safety and risks liability for the hospital and its emergency department staff.

In some states statutes creating and regulating government hospitals include provisions that deal with procedures for patient discharge. Statutory provisions in several states apply to nongovernment hospitals. Discharge provisions are ordinarily general in nature and define the right to discharge a patient as an act of discretion by the managing hospital authorities, based on the patient's medical condition or on other suitable reasons. Most discharge statutes merely provide that rules may be promulgated for discharging patients. The legal principles regarding discharge have generally derived from court decisions and do not seem to vary on the basis of the hospital's ownership.

The general rule is that a patient should be discharged only upon the written order of a physician who is familiar with the patient's condition. Patients unable to care for themselves, such as infants or aged or disabled patients, should be discharged only in the custody of relatives, friends, or agents of government or private social welfare agencies. Discharge of a patient apparently unable to reach home safely because of age or disability could constitute negligence if such a patient met with an injury on leaving the hospital. The appropriate standard of care may require that the hospital provide or arrange a suitable escort for such a patient. After a discharge order has been given by the physician, the hospital no longer need permit the patient to remain except to ensure that such necessary assistance is provided. If the patient refuses to leave the premises, he or she is in the status of a trespasser, and reasonable force may be used to secure his or her removal. It would appear that the aid of police might be sought in the event that such a person must be forced to depart.

In emergency department situations, persons may be hesitant to leave for a variety of reasons. It is important for the staff to discuss with patients the reasons for their hesitancy to be certain a patient is not discharged inappropriately.

In addition to the problem raised by patients who hesitate to leave upon discharge, there is the problem of patients who wish to leave against medical advice. When it is clear to the emergency department staff that, for specified reasons, it is unwise for a patient to leave, every effort should be made to convince that patient to stay. Patients may wish to leave for a variety of reasons. Some of the reasons may be very personal—for example, a single parent who feels the need to return home to children left in someone else's care.

If every attempt made to encourage the patient to remain has failed, there is no recourse but to let the patient leave. In this situation, the patient should be requested to sign a form that acknowledges he or she is leaving the hospital against advice (see Exhibit 7-1). Whenever possible, it would be wise for the responsible physician to handle this matter, so the patient can be informed about alternatives and the risks involved in leaving. If for any reason the patient refuses to sign the form, this fact plus the time the patient left should be noted in the hospital record. Also, any other pertinent information such as the reasons given for leaving against advice, the persons who accompanied the patient home, any statements the patient made as to plans to obtain other care, and the patient's destination other than home should be recorded.

Exhibit 7-1 Form for Patients Who Leave the Hospital Against Medical Advice

---

LEAVING HOSPITAL AGAINST MEDICAL ADVICE

Date_____

I certify that (I) (_____) a
                          Name, if other than signer
patient in the _____ hospital (am) (is) leaving the hospital against the advice of the attending physician and the hospital administrators. Dr. _____ explained to me my
                    (Named Physician)
condition as _____ and my refusal to continue treatment will result in _____ and will seriously affect my life and chances for regaining normal health.

The hospital suggested that if treatment has not been satisfactory, it should be sought immediately at another institution.

I hereby release the hospital, its nurses and employees, together with all physicians in any way connected with me as a patient, from liability for any ill effects which may result from this action. I have read this form and understand its meaning.

(In the event the patient, or the parent or guardian in the case of a minor patient, refuses to sign the form, this fact should be noted on the form, and the form placed in the patient's record.)

_____
(Signature)

_____
(Relationship)

_____
(Witness)

Clearly, the emergency department policy and procedure manual should include a section on patients who leave against advice. The manual should also address the problem of patients who refuse to leave when discharged. It is essential that the staff adhere to such policies and procedures. These should be amended regularly to address current practice.

ABANDONMENT

Emergency department physicians must always be concerned about the problem of legal abandonment in the premature or inappropriate discharge of a patient. Legally abandonment refers to the termination of the physician-patient relationship by the physician without the patient's consent. It also implies that the patient has not been given sufficient time or opportunity to obtain the services of another physician. Thus it is essential that upon discharge the emergency department physician give the patient clear and specific instructions on the follow-up care that is recommended. The patient should understand these instructions and should not be discharged until it is clear that the instructions are understood. Any instructions given should be in writing, and a copy should be put into the hospital record. If the patient does not comprehend English, an interpreter is needed. Use the hospital interpreter or an English-speaking relative or friend.

The instruction sheet should be signed by the patient. This constitutes some protection should the patient later charge the emergency room physician with abandonment. To provide even better protection, the instruction sheet should always advise the patient to return to the emergency department if complications arise. Thus, the emergency room physician will have made the emergency room available for later problems.

A recurring problem in many emergency departments involves patients who are treated, return home and have a recurrence of symptoms, feel worse, develop complications from the treatment or medication, and phone in for advice. In this sort of situation, the patient should be instructed to return to the emergency department for additional treatment. Patients should not be put off because they've called at an inconvenient hour or because their problem does not sound serious. If the patient is refused treatment and suffers as a result, the emergency department risks liability for both negligence and abandonment. This is especially true if the patient has been advised to call again in the morning or return to the department at that time, because it effectively precludes the patient from seeking alternative forms of care.

STATUTORY PROVISIONS FOR DISCHARGE

In some states, statutes creating and regulating government hospitals include provisions that deal with procedures for the discharge of patients. In several states there are statutory provisions that apply to nongovernment hospitals. Discharge provisions are ordinarily an act of discretion on the part of the managing authorities, based on the patient's medical condition or other suitable criteria. Thus the discharge section of the statute governing the Colorado General Hospital, a government hospital, provides as follows:

§ 124-4-9. Discharge of Patients.

(1) Whenever in the opinion of the superintendent of the hospital, any patient should be discharged therefrom as cured, or as no longer needing treatment, or for other good and sufficient reasons, said superintendent shall discharge said patient.

(2) If, upon the discharge of any patient from the hospital, it shall appear to the superintendent thereof that said patient, upon his discharge, is not financially able to provide himself with transportation to his home or other place to which he may be discharged, said superintendent may authorize the payment of such transportation on behalf of said patient.

Colo. Rev. Stat. Ann. § 124-4-9 (1964).

Other state statutes have similar provisions, making a discharge a discretionary act. Provisions of this type set out the same considerations that hospitals in general would ordinarily consider when deciding whether or not to discharge a patient. Thus, in the Colorado statute, the hospital superintendent may discharge a patient (1) when that patient is cured; (2) when that patient is no longer in need of treatment; (3) when treatment can no longer benefit that patient's case; and (4) for other good and sufficient reasons.

Most discharge statutes merely provide that rules may be promulgated for discharging patients. Thus, clearly, it is incumbent on hospital emergency departments to formulate discharge policies that protect both the hospital and the patient. In the case of litigation on a question of inappropriate discharge, the matter will, by and large, have to be handled by the courts.

DISCHARGE OF PATIENTS IN NEED OF FURTHER CARE

As stated earlier in this chapter, when a hospital undertakes to treat a person, it must not act unreasonably in removing that person from the premises. The law requires that a patient be kept in the hospital and that treatment be continued if it is foreseeable that his or her condition would be aggravated or the risks of danger increased by removal.

In the leading New York case of *Meiselman* v. *Crown Heights Hospital,* 285 N.Y. 389, 34 N.E. 2d 367 (1941), a child undergoing treatment for osteomyelitis was discharged by the defendant hospital—this despite the fact that both of the child's legs were in casts, open wounds were draining through windows in the plaster casts, and he was still suffering a high temperature. The child's father was assured that no further hospitalization was required and that any care necessary could be given at home under the direction and supervision of the chief of the hospital's surgical staff. The home care was unsatisfactory and the child's condition deteriorated. This led to his hospitalization at another institution. At the time of the trial, the child was crippled. The basis of the suit was the wrongful discharge of the child, when it should have been apparent that his condition would probably deteriorate. That the hospital bill was partly unpaid at the time of discharge was taken by the court to indicate that the hospital's overriding interest was financial. Because the child's physical condition was not given primary consideration, the discharge was seen as *prima facie* unreasonable.

Another case revolved around the issue of child abuse. In *Landeros* v. *Flood,* 131 Cal. Rptr. 69, 551 P. 2d 389 (1976), the California Supreme Court ruled a hospital liable for subsequent injuries sustained by a battered child who was improperly released to the care of her parents. In this case, an 11-month-old child who appeared to be physically abused charged (through her guardian ad litem) both the facility at which she was treated and one of its physicians with negligently failing to order x-rays or report her condition to the police or the juvenile probation department as required by state law. Because "battered child syndrome" has become an accepted medical diagnosis, the court ruled it was proper for the patient to show by expert testimony that the physician should have known how to diagnose and treat this condition.

In addition, the court ruled that the physician's and hospital's exculpatory claim that they had not legally caused the patient's injuries subsequent to their examination of her was without merit. Rather, it reasoned, the patient was entitled to prove that it was reasonably foreseeable at the time of her release that her parents were likely to resume their physical abuse.

In *Kroupa* v. *Southampton Hospital,* 374 N.Y.S. 2d 37 (1975), the patient, a minor, was brought by his father to the emergency room of the hospital suffering from violent stomach pains and nausea. Later the same day the child was discharged from the hospital. Ten days later the patient was readmitted to the hospital in critical condition with a ruptured appendix. The father brought action charging the hospital with negligence both in diagnosing the illness and in discharging the child when he was in need of further attention. The hospital attempted to bar its liability on the basis of the father's lack of parental discretion in not seeking aid between the time of discharge and readmission. The court found that the son had no recognizable tort action against his father which the hospital could use to bar its liability or as a basis for repayment from the father.

The North Carolina Court of Appeals took a similar position in allowing a mother to recover damages for the death of her three-year-old daughter. The jury found the plaintiff's intestate death was caused by the defendant's negligence, as alleged in the complaint, and awarded damages of $65,000. In *Spillman* v. *Forsyth Memorial Hospital,* 30 N.C.A. 406, 227 S.E. 2d 292 (1976), damages were awarded after it was demonstrated that the staff of a hospital emergency room was negligent in the way it provided medical treatment to the child.

At the time the mother brought her daughter to the hospital emergency room, in May 1968, the child's stomach and navel were swollen, her temperature registered 105 degrees F, and she was vomiting and screaming in pain. Upon examination by the emergency room physician, she was given some "red looking medicine" but was not admitted to the hospital. X-rays and blood and urine samples were not taken. The next night, after the child's condition failed to improve, the mother returned with her daughter to the emergency room. The emergency room physician first called the mother's attention to a posted sign stating that welfare patients had to go to the clinic. Then the physician examined the child once again and sent her home. When mother and child returned the following day, the child was treated immediately with oxygen and other measures, but she died within 30 minutes. On autopsy the pathologist listed the cause of death as peritonitis due to, or as a consequence of, a perforated appendix of an estimated four days' duration. He testified that the child had acute gangrenous appendicitis, which he defined as "a far advanced infection in the appendix." Medical experts testified that the failure to admit and treat the child "was not standard acceptable medical treatment" in that community or in similar communities in this country.

The three cases just described indicate that emergency department staff must be extremely careful to not discharge patients prematurely because such premature discharge could result in risk to a patient's health and safety.

Compare these cases to the traditional rule on admittance stated first in *Birmingham Baptist Hospital* v. *Crews,* 229 Ala. 398, 157 So. 224 (1934). In this Alabama case (discussed more fully in Chapter 3) a child suffering from diphtheria was brought to the emergency department of a charitable hospital.

The house physician rendered treatment—consisting of swabbing the child's throat, administering oxygen, and giving injections of anti-toxin—and the child's father was informed that the hospital did not accept patients with contagious diseases. The child was returned home by automobile and died soon after.

In the suit the parents contended that the child's death was accelerated by the weakening effect of the anti-toxin on her heart, coupled with the exertion of the trip home. It was urged that, after the hospital had commenced emergency treatment, it was obliged to render ordinary hospital services and should not have told the child's father to take her away.

The hospital was held not liable because the court found that no duty existed to accept the patient.

> Defendant is a private corporation, and not a public institution, and owes the public no duty to accept any patient not desired by it. In this respect it is not similar to a public utility. It is not necessary to assign any reason for its refusal to accept a patient for hospital service.
> *Birmingham Baptist Hospital* v. *Crews,* 157 So. 224, 225.

The opinion further stated, after pointing out that the hospital's rules prohibited the admission of contagious disease patients,

> We think that such treatment [the emergency care rendered] does not justify an inference that defendant undertook to render ordinary hospital service in violation of its rules, so as to endanger the life or health of other patients.

> To uphold plaintiff's contention, we assume that, if defendant did not propose to render hospital service, it should have sent the child away in a desperate condition without emergency treatment, when such treatment was available and provided the only hope of recovery. The willingness of defendant to provide such treatment should not be used to its prejudice for not violating its rules and endangering other patients.

The *Crews* case illustrates the traditional view that a person does not possess a positive right to be admitted to a hospital. However, the court also recognized the distinction between the traditional view and the principle that the exercise of control might give rise to a duty on the part of the hospital to meet the appropriate standard of care. The court is reluctant, on the facts of this case, to require the hospital to admit everyone, under all circumstances, in need of hospital care merely because emergency assistance is rendered. Such a requirement might conceivably inhibit hospitals from furnishing any emergency care due to fear of liability.

The courts initially view a hospital and a prospective patient in much the same manner they view two ordinary persons. Thus the preceding principles may be formulated as a rule providing that an individual has no right to aid from another individual or a hospital. However, if control is exercised, neither an individual nor a hospital can defend unreasonable conduct on the grounds that it had no duty to act. Rather, the duty can only be discharged by conduct in accord with the appropriate standard of care.

The appropriate standard of care was an important issue in a Texas case, *Garcia* v. *Memorial Hospital,* 557 S.W. 2d 859 (1977). The facts in this case reveal that the infant child, Richard Garcia, was taken to the emergency room of the defendant hospital late at night, suffering from difficulty in breathing. The emergency room nurse on duty contacted a local physician by phone. Over the phone and without seeing the child, the physician ordered medication and instructed the parents to return home with the child and observe him carefully there. At 7:30 a.m., the child was brought back to the hospital and, this time, admitted. Nevertheless, the infant died, due to aspiration of vomitus and mucous filling the lungs, because the hospital's lack of a pediatric endotracheal tube prevented proper treatment.

The parents brought a wrongful death action against the hospital and two of its employees. The court rendered summary judgment for the hospital and the employees based on the defendant's claim of governmental immunity (as the hospital was a subdivision of the State of Texas). The parents appealed this decision. The Court of Appeals reversed the judgment of the county district court and remanded the case for a new trial, holding that a complaint alleging that the defendants were negligent (due to failure to ensure that the vital component of necessary life-sustaining equipment would be available and ready for use) stated a cause of action under the Texas Tort Claims Act. Thus, in this act of negligence, the appropriate standard of care was not met. The court expected a hospital emergency department to be adequately staffed and supplied with life-saving equipment as are other similar hospital emergency departments. The court held that the negligent failure to furnish a pediatric endotracheal tube brought the case within the statutory waiver of immunity.

The appellate court did not address the issue of medical orders by phone, but one can predict that this issue would be raised in the new trial.

In *Bourgeois* v. *Dade County,* 99 S. 2d 575 (Fla. Sup. Ct., 1957), suit was brought alleging negligence in emergency room care. The facts in this case reveal that Nicholas Geoffrey Bourgeois was found unconscious in front of a hotel, stretched out on the lawn, at about 1:50 a.m. on a September night in

1954. The police called an ambulance, and Bourgeois was taken on a stretcher to Jackson Memorial Hospital.

Bourgeois was taken into the hospital emergency room. The intern testified in court that Bourgeois was not unconscious on admission, although he was incoherent. The intern did not attempt to take a history and did not take x-rays. After performing a relatively superficial clinical examination, the intern released the man to a nurse for return to the hospital police room for delivery to the police as a drunk. The intern testified that the man's breath literally reeked of alcohol. The police officer who called for an ambulance had detected a "slight odor" of alcohol. The ambulance driver noticed none at all.

The police picked up Bourgeois at about 3 a.m. He was taken to the municipal jail in a patrol car. The police officer testified that Bourgeois slumped over on the seat of the automobile as if his "back were broken." He was put into a cell where he was found dead at 7 a.m. Death was caused by air and hemorrhaging in the thoracic cavity, resulting from the piercing of the cavity by broken ribs.

Because it was felt that the evidence of causal connection between the alleged negligence and the ultimate death was too speculative to justify consideration by a jury, the trial judge directed a verdict for the defendant. An appeal was brought to the Supreme Court of Florida. The court stated:

> Admittedly the science of medicine is not an exact science. Physicians are not to be held liable for honest errors of judgment. . . . To hold one liable it must be shown that the course which he pursued was clearly against the course recognized as correct by his profession.
>
> . . . The responsibility and degree of care imposed upon the . . . hospital is to be measured by the responsibility and degree of care imposed upon its employees, the intern and nurses in the emergency ward.
>
> Here it appears that a man, dressed only in shorts, was delivered into the custody of the emergency room attendants at about 2:00 a.m. by an ambulance driver. Although the intern testified that the man was belligerent and reeking with alcohol, both the police officer who found him and the ambulance driver who delivered him testified that at most there was only a mild odor of alcohol and the man breathed heavily but did not utter a word. After fifteen or twenty minutes the intern discharged the patient as a drunk. The factual problem is whether he should have pursued a more thorough course of inquiry and examination under the circumstances. No history of the man's condition or the facts leading up to his delivery to the hospital was at any time obtained. No X-rays were made. The hospital director

himself testified that if a patient was unconscious and unable, as distinguished from unwilling, to give his name and state how he was injured when delivered to the hospital, then releasing him in the same condition would in his judgment fall below the standard of care required under the circumstances. The physician who was the supervisor of the emergency room at the time testified that if a patient in the condition of Bourgeois were admitted and could not give a history of his condition, and one could not be obtained, then he would certainly take X-rays in an effort to form a diagnosis. He also testified that he had seen Bourgeois when he was admitted to the hospital, that he could not say that the man was intoxicated and that the fact that he had a normal pulse rate was inconsistent with a state of intoxication.

Bourgeois v. *Dade County,* 99 So. 2d 575, 577.

The court held that in view of the contradictory testimony about the patient's sobriety and consciousness, and in view of all the circumstances reflected in the record, there was adequate evidence of negligence in the treatment, examination, and ultimate diagnosis of the decedent's condition to justify taking the case to the jury.

It can be seen from this case that a cursory examination leading to the discharge of a patient who later dies will expose the hospital and the emergency department to liability for negligence.

In *Niles* v. *City of San Rafael,* 42 Cal. App. 230, 116 Cal. Rptr. 733 (1974), a suit was brought for discharge without adequate treatment. The jury awarded the plaintiffs $4,025,000, of which the doctor and the hospital were to pay $4 million. In this case, an 11-year-old child, Kelly Niles, was injured during a fight while playing softball at a school playground. Kelly's father brought him to the emergency room of Mt. Zion Hospital in San Francisco, where he was examined by two nurses, an intern, and a pediatric resident. Kelly had sustained a small fracture of the skull that tore an artery. The resulting bleeding between the dura and the skull caused an accumulation of clotted blood that generated severe pressure on the brain. The intern determined that Kelly should be admitted; the nurses and the resident physician agreed. The resident physician, who was the intern's supervisor, marked Kelly's chart "Admit."

After the resident had concurred in the intern's recommendation that Kelly be admitted, someone in the admitting office incorrectly told the intern that Kelly could not be admitted because he was not being treated by a private physician who enjoyed staff privileges at the hospital. The resident sought help in gaining admittance for Kelly from the director of the pediatric outpatient clinic. Dr. Haskins, the director, discharged the boy in the care of his father.

When a child with a possible head injury was released from the emergency room, it was the hospital's usual practice to give the parent a sheet listing symptoms that indicated the child should be returned to the hospital. The head injury sheet used in the emergency room of Mt. Zion Hospital listed seven symptoms, five of which were present when Kelly was released from the hospital. The sheet was not given to Kelly's father.

Kelly's father took the child home. From a first aid book he learned that a slowing pulse rate is indicative of bleeding within the skull. When Kelly's pulse rate fell and one pupil dilated, his father rushed him back to the emergency room.

Surgery was performed to remove a blood clot and the bleeding was stopped. However, Kelly was in a coma for 46 days following surgery, and he suffered irreparable brain damage.

On appeal, the medical defendant attacked the judgment as excessive. The court found that the jury had adequate evidence to sustain its finding of $4 million against the medical defendants and $25,000 against the city and school district. The plaintiffs had introduced evidence at the trial to support the composition of the verdict.

This was a tragic and unfortunate case for everyone involved. One error compounded another, resulting in permanent disability for a formerly healthy child. Clearly, the child was discharged prematurely and inappropriately, aggravating his condition and risking his health and safety.

REFUSAL TO DISCHARGE

A distinctly different problem from premature or inappropriate discharge is refusal to discharge. In this area the usual problems seen by the courts involve persons with mental conditions and problems related to payment of the hospital bill.

A patient of sound mind who desires to leave a hospital may not be prevented from leaving. Such conduct would constitute false imprisonment. In order to maintain an action for false imprisonment, a person must show that there was an actual confinement or restraint, either by means of physical barriers or by threats that intimidated the individual into compliance and placed her or him in reasonable apprehension of harm. It must also be shown that the defendant intended to confine the aggrieved person. Unlike negligence, no actual damage must be proved; the law assumes harm has resulted.

Thus a hospital may not detain a patient against his or her will for failure to pay the hospital bill. In *Gadsden General Hospital* v. *Hamilton,* 212 Ala. 531, 103 So. 553 (1925), it was held that a patient, detained against her will for 11 hours by an order that she could not leave the hospital until her bill was paid, could recover damages for false imprisonment. The court said: "The fact that plaintiff's bill . . . had not been paid, afforded no sort of excuse for detaining plaintiff against her will."

In *Hoffman* v. *Clinic Hospital,* 213 N.C. 669, 197 S.E. 161 (1938), an action for false imprisonment was brought by a patient against a charitable hospital. The plaintiff alleged that she was forbidden to leave until her bill was paid. The court, in discussing the facts, found that no force or threat of force had been used and that the patient could not have been in reasonable apprehension of force being used. Her belief that she could not leave without paying her bill was insufficient to constitute an unlawful detention. However, the *Hoffman* case recognized that if force or the threat of force had been used to prevent a patient from leaving, the conduct would have been actionable.

A hospital was held liable for detaining an infant patient in *Bedard* v. *Notre Dame Hospital,* 89 R. I. 195, 151 A. 2d 690 (1959), where the hospital refused to discharge the child unless the hospital bill was paid. The mother had been notified that treatment had been completed, and she was ready to accept custody of the child. The court stated that custody of a minor child is a legally protected interest and that interference with the parent's right to custody is an actionable wrong.

In addition to situations involving unpaid bills, there are other circumstances in which hospitals may not desire to discharge patients. However, the fact that hospital personnel believe that it is medically unwise for a patient to leave does not grant that hospital an absolute right to prevent the patient from leaving.

In *Smith* v. *Henry Ford Hospital,* an unreported Michigan case, Mr. Smith voluntarily requested and was granted admission into the defendant hospital. Because he was suffering from heart disease, he was placed in the coronary unit. Upon improvement he was transferred to a semiprivate room. The other patient in the room was "very elderly and out of contact with reality." Mr. Smith liked neither the room nor the other patient and decided to leave. Two orderlies and two nurses' aides physically returned him to his room over his protest, although no rough treatment was used. He was tied down with a belt 12 feet long. Mr. Smith escaped from the belt, tied the belt to the other patient's bed, and attempted to escape by sliding down the belt from his second-story room. But the belt was too short, and he was injured when he fell to the ground.

There was no claim by the hospital that Mr. Smith was mentally unsound. The court awarded him damages for the injury sustained in the attempted escape, resulting from the false imprisonment and the assault and battery.

The risk to the patient's well-being, should he or she leave the hospital, must be made apparent to the patient, and it would be entirely proper for hospital personnel to urge that the patient reconsider the decision to leave. However, the patient should not be prevented from leaving either by actual physical restraint or threat of force. Keeping a patient in a hospital against his or her will for the purpose of rendering treatment will give rise to a cause of action in much the same manner as an unauthorized surgical procedure. In both instances, the hospital is acting against the patient's will. And clearly, in both instances, the law will not permit such conduct.

Where the patient seeking discharge is of unsound mind and there exists a substantial risk of danger to his or her life or the lives of others, the hospital is permitted to prevent the patient's departure, using such physical restraint as is reasonable under the circumstances. However, it should be noted that the hospital is not privileged to use any more force than is necessary to effect this restraint successfully. In such situations, statutory procedures to commit such a patient to a mental institution should be instituted promptly. The confinement of a mentally ill patient is privileged only when there is good reason to believe there exists a danger to the patient or to the lives of others. Mental illness alone is not sufficient reason to make restraint legally proper. For example, patients may be psychotic and clearly out of touch with reality, yet present no threat to themselves or others.

If a patient who is suffering from a contagious disease desires to leave, the hospital has the right to restrain him or her until the local public health authorities are informed and given the opportunity to take action to protect the community. There has been legal support for the hospital's right to exercise a duty to prevent mentally ill persons who are dangerous to themselves or others or persons afflicted with communicable diseases from leaving the hospital premises. The hospital may thus be required to act in order to prevent imposition of liability if such persons harm others.

Cases of false imprisonment of psychiatric patients have been reported. In *Marcus* v. *Liebman,* No. 76-286 (Cook County Cir. Ct., 1978), a psychiatric patient who voluntarily entered a hospital for bedrest withdrew her request to be discharged following a staff physician's warning that he could commit her to a mental facility if she refused to remain hospitalized. In response to the patient's allegation that she was thereby subject to false imprisonment, the physician countered that it was unreasonable for her to believe that she was not free to leave. Given the patient's poor "mental condition, however, and the fact that she was behind locked hospital doors," an Illinois appellate court decided that a jury should rule whether the physician's warning and her continued hospitalization constituted "false imprisonment."

In *Johnson* v. *United States,* 547 F. 2d 688 (D.C. Cir., 1976), the U.S. Court of Appeals for the District of Columbia dismissed false imprisonment and medical malpractice claims against a veterans' administration hospital. The claims had been brought by a patient who was committed to a public psychiatric hospital following the emergency application of a VA hospital staff physician. The patient contended that the VA physician failed to use standard medical practice in seeking his commitment, a charge the court specifically rejected.

The VA physician, the court stated, clearly satisfied his statutory duty as spelled out in the law. Moreover, it observed, the patient had not been confined on the VA physician's application but on the certificate of the admitting hospital's psychiatrist, who after examining the patient, determined that he required "detention and observation." The commitment statute, the court noted, specifically allows:

> a physician "who has reason to believe that [his patient] is mentally ill and, because of the illness, is likely to injure himself or others if he is not immediately detained" is statutorily empowered, without a warrant, "[to] take the [patient] into custody, transport him to a public or private hospital, and make application for his admission thereto for purposes of emergency observation and diagnosis." The only additional requirement which the statute imposes upon the physician is that "[the] application shall reveal the circumstances under which the person was taken into custody and the reasons therefor."
>
> D.C. Code § 21-521 (1973).

In relying on statutory provisions for emergency admission of patients requiring psychiatric care, emergency department staff should try to ensure that the provisions are not violated in the process. In *Sukeforth* v. *Thegen,* 256 A. 2d 162 (1969), the plaintiff was brought to a mental hospital for an examination so as to certify insanity. Defendant physician, without seeing or examining the plaintiff, issued a certificate that he had examined the plaintiff, that in his opinion the plaintiff was mentally ill, and that because of said illness the plaintiff was likely to injure himself if not restrained immediately. Based on this certificate, the plaintiff was taken into custody and confined for three days at a state hospital. In a complaint for false imprisonment, the defendant's motion to dismiss was granted.

The plaintiff appealed, relying on common law for recovery, citing precedent that held that all those who by direct act or indirect procurement personally participate in or proximately cause a false imprisonment or unlawful detention are liable. The defendant relied on a statute providing for emergency admittance to a hospital, which grants immunity to physicians from civil liability when acting in a quasi-judicial capacity.

The court defined the issue presented as whether the defendant physician enjoyed such protective immunity under the facts alleged, when immunity would not otherwise be available to an ordinary person who was guilty of like conduct.

The court held that no physician acting in a quasi-judicial capacity can reasonably expect the protection of immunity if that physician had not seen fit to perform the elementary act—the examination—by which he or she acquires jurisdiction over the person restrained. To omit the examination, the court reasoned, and thereafter falsely certify that the examination had in fact been made and an opinion reached as a result of it, is more than a failure to perform a jurisdictional act. It is a matter that shocks the conscience and scarcely accords with the high standards of the medical profession, the court said. In conclusion, the court noted that there must be some form of personal observation by the physician as circumstances may permit, in which case the jurisdictional requirement of the statute would be satisfied. But to base a judgment as to the presence of a mental illness exclusively upon reports and observations of others is certainly short of the jurisdictional requirements, and the physician would therefore not be insulated from civil liability under the statute. The appeal was sustained and the case remanded for further proceeding.

Occasionally, the emergency department staff sees cases where the threat of harm to self or others by a person is seen as a threat to the staff. In *Fish* v. *Regents of the University of California,* 246 Cal. 2d 327, 54 Cal. Rptr. 656 (1966), the plaintiff brought his father to the Mission Emergency Hospital after he had applied sunlamp treatment to his father's bedsores. Believing his father suffered severe burns as a result of the treatment, the plaintiff berated the physicians at the hospital after being told that the burns were not the father's main difficulty. One of the nurses reported that the plaintiff, having left the hospital, threatened to shoot himself or someone else. The plaintiff then phoned one of the doctors, saying he was on his way back to the hospital and "wanted to make sure" that the doctor was still there. Because the doctor was fearful for his life, hospital security apprehended the plaintiff. The physician who had been threatened then consulted with another physician. That physician had the plaintiff detained for observation. A complete notation of the sequence of events was made in the hospital record. After several days of observation, one of the physicians in the psychopathic ward concluded that a mental illness petition should be filed in Superior Court. Medical examiners from the Superior Court found the plaintiff suffering from a paranoid personality but found no reason sufficient for commitment. The plaintiff then sued for malicious prosecution and false imprisonment.

After disposing of the action for malicious prosecution, holding that various statutes produced immunity for this public entity, the court found that in absence of evidence that the threatened physician acted in bad faith or took an active part in detaining the plaintiff, the doctor and regents of the university could not be held liable for false imprisonment.

The court recognized the threatened physician's inability to order detention of the plaintiff, as he was a general surgeon. The consulting psychopathic ward physician had the discretionary responsibility of making a good faith judgment, weighing the obligation to protect the threatened physician and other persons against the personal rights and liberty of the plaintiff. The hospital produced enough evidence to demonstrate good faith and reasonable judgment. In addition, there was a statute providing immunity to the city and county for the diagnosis of a mental illness, and this was held to include a preliminary diagnosis.

This case shows the importance the court accorded the facts. That the hospital had enough evidence to demonstrate good faith and reasonable judgment weighed heavily in the hospital's ability to avoid liability. Thus it is essential that emergency room staff members have clear policies and procedures to accommodate the psychiatric management of persons who might have to be detained against their will. Because state statutes on emergency commitment vary, a copy of the law should be in the procedure manual and its provisions should be adhered to carefully.

In some emergency departments this may be a common problem; in others it may be a rare occurrence. An emergency commitment for mental illness seriously limits a person's freedom, and it is an action not to be undertaken lightly. Other possible alternatives should be exhausted before instituting proceedings for emergency commitment.

ESCAPES AND ELOPEMENTS

The common law rule is that one person owes no duty to control the conduct of another. However, two exceptions to this rule have generally been recognized: (1) when the defendant stands in some special relationship to either the person whose conduct needs to be controlled or to the foreseeable victim of the conduct; (2) where the defendant has engaged or undertaken to engage in affirmative action to control the anticipated dangerous conduct of a person or to protect the prospective victim (Rest. 2d Torts, 1965 §§ 321-324a). Both relationships give rise to affirmative duties for the benefit of third parties and have been found to impose liability on hospitals for failing to admit, or for improperly releasing or discharging patients with mental disorders or communicable diseases, or for failing to warn the community of a patient's dangerous condition. The majority of these cases, however, do not involve the emergency department of general hospitals.

In *Torres* v. *City of New York,* 396 N.Y.S. 2d 34 (App. Div., 1977), aff. 58 N.Y. App. Div. 647 (1977), a case that did involve the emergency department of a general hospital, a New York appellate court ruled that a hospital was not liable for injuries suffered by a patient who walked away from an emergency room shortly after his admission and thereafter jumped in front of a subway train. The patient was taken to the hospital by a police officer and left unattended in the emergency room, contrary to the hospital's standard procedure. As a result of the jump in front of the subway train, he suffered injuries necessitating the amputation of his right leg. However, the court concluded that no legal ground existed to prevent the patient from leaving or to require that the nurse in the emergency room should have restrained the patient, and no testimony in court indicated a deviation from good hospital practice.

In cases where there seems to be reasonable cause to believe a patient may cause harm to self or others, the emergency department staff should make every effort to detain the patient voluntarily for self-protection and the protection of others. Every effort should be made to contact family, friends, and anyone else who could possibly reason with the patient, including social workers, the clergy, and sympathetic staff members. An attempt at psychiatric consultation should be made if such consultation is available.

Sometimes all these attempts are made to no avail. Sometimes it is almost useless to try because the patient is overdosed on drugs, inebriated, or comatose from a suicide attempt. In cases where every alternative has been tried but has failed, statutory emergency commitment should always be viewed as a last resort, to be used only to protect persons from harming themselves or others. The policy and procedure manual detailing the commitment procedure should be very clear on what situations warrant such a drastic measure.

PART IV

Laws and Regulations

Chapter 8

Reporting Laws

In order to promote the detection and appropriate action by public officials in cases involving the safety and health of the community, a number of states have enacted a series of reporting laws. These laws typically require reports to be made to specified officials, provide for the confidential handling of those reports, and protect those who make the reports in good faith from civil and criminal liability. The list of laws will vary from state to state, and some will affect hospitals in differing degrees. Some of the common types of reporting laws relate to child abuse and neglect, elderly abuse and neglect, gunshot and other violent wounds, rape, abortion, poisoning, venereal disease, specified communicable diseases, tuberculosis, cancer, drug abuse, and all suspicious or unattended deaths.

In *Whalen* v. *Roe,* 429 U.S. 589 (1977), an unsuccessful challenge was made to New York's requirement for reporting detailed patient information to a computerized data system whenever Schedule II drugs (for example, codeine, morphine) are prescribed or dispensed. The courts have upheld these mandatory reporting laws over an individual's right to privacy when the state can show a compelling and overriding interest and has taken sufficient steps to maintain appropriate confidentiality and limited use of the data collected.

The reporting laws can be ignored only at the hospital's peril. A California case, *Landeros* v. *Flood,* 131 Cal. Rptr. 69, 551 P. 2d 389 (Cal. Sup. Ct., 1976), held a hospital liable for failing to report child abuse when lack of intervention resulted in further injuries to the child.

The staff members of emergency departments must be aware of the reporting requirements in the states in which they practice. Indeed, with the increasing use of emergency rooms by the general public (as discussed in Chapter 2), it becomes more and more important for emergency personnel to familiarize themselves with reporting laws and to follow them. Although the number and kind of situations seen will vary depending on the size and location of the emergency department, there is little doubt that few, if any, emergency rooms can afford to ignore reporting laws. This is not only because such laws are important to the general health and welfare of the people and because they will be upheld by the courts, but because so many of the reportable diseases and injuries are seen with great frequency in emergency rooms. Cases of child abuse, elderly abuse, venereal disease, and drug abuse and addiction are examples of situations seen more commonly in the emergency department than in other departments of the general hospital. This is also true of situations resulting from violence, including cases of assault with a deadly weapon and attempts at self-destruction.

The governing board of each general hospital maintaining an emergency department, together with the emergency department personnel, should address the issue of reportable incidents in the emergency department policy and procedure manual. What is included in this manual, and in what detail, will be governed by the applicable state and federal laws together with the internal rules of the hospital. The policies and procedures should clearly and carefully reflect the general practice of the emergency room. As certain situations are seen with more or less frequency, the policies should be amended to address current practice. Policies should also be amended to reflect changes in reporting laws.

REPORTABLE DISEASES

In all the states there are public health laws and regulations that require the reporting of specific diseases. Some of these diseases are rarely seen in any part of this country. For example, Hansen's Disease, more commonly called leprosy, is rarely seen in emergency departments anywhere in the United States. Rocky Mountain Spotted Fever is a reportable disease seen with little frequency in the eastern part of the country; it is more common in the western states. Tuberculosis is a reportable disease seen with less and less frequency across the country, whereas venereal disease is being seen with increasing frequency in all parts of the country.

Public health departments usually specify that reportable diseases be recorded on form cards. The physician who has established the diagnosis is most often held legally responsible for completing the form card. In some cases of highly contagious diseases, such as smallpox and yellow fever, the reporting laws and regulations require that state public health officials be notified immediately by phone or telegraph. However, in the case of other reportable diseases, regulations usually provide that the form cards be submitted to the local health officer. This is power delegated from the state health officer to the local health officer.

Often the statutes or regulations specify that the responsibility for reporting communicable diseases falls on persons other than physicians. For example, a New York regulation provides:

> SANITARY CODE, Ch. 1, Sec. 2.12 (1973). Reporting by others than physicians of cases or diseases presumably communicable.
>
> When no physician is in attendance it shall be the duty of the head of a private household or the person in charge of any institution, school, motel, boarding house, camp or vessel or any public health nurse or any other person having actual knowledge of an individual affected with any disease presumably communicable, to report immediately the name and address of such person to the local health officer. Until official action on such case has been taken, strict isolation shall be maintained.

Statutes requiring the reporting of communicable diseases emphasize the need for such statutes. If the state is to protect its citizens' health through its power to quarantine, the state must have developed procedures ensuring the prompt reporting of infection or disease. Thus statutes and regulations often require reporting by persons other than and in addition to the physician establishing the diagnosis.

Because the emergency room is sometimes the scene of birth, emergency room personnel should be cognizant of the requirements that govern the reporting of diseases in newborns. Many states require anyone in attendance at birth to report, either to the physician in charge or to an appropriate health officer, all instances of diarrhea, staphylococcal disease, or other infections. Most states provide for penalizing any violator of these laws.

In particular, health personnel must report inflammation, swelling, redness, or unnatural discharge from an infant's eyes. The Rhode Island statute is typical:

> § 23-13-6. REPORTS OF OPHTHALMIA NEONATORUM. It shall be the duty of any physician, midwife, nurse, parent or other person or persons assisting in the care of any infant to report within twelve (12) hours after noting the same, any such case of ophthalmia neonatorum coming to his or her attention, to the department of health.

Statutory reporting requirements are made under each state's police power. In addition to the fact that the state is interested in maintaining the health of its citizens, a state requires reporting and treating of ophthalmia neonatorum because public funds might have to be used to train or care for blind children.

Phenylketonuria (PKU) is one of the most recent additions to the list of reportable conditions for newborns. Actually, here the chief purpose of the reporting requirements is to encourage the testing and treatment of infants for PKU. Some statutes, such as Louisiana's, require a report to an appropriate health agency if tests reveal PKU in an infant. Louisiana also has a similar requirement concerning sickle cell anemia:

Part XV. Phenylketonuria: Meniscocytosis § 1299.1 Tests

A.   The physician attending a newborn child, or the person attending a newborn child that was not attended by a physician, shall cause said child to be subjected to a phenylketonuria test that has been approved by the State Department of Public Health, provided, however, no such test shall be given to any child whose parents object thereto. If the test is positive the attending physician or person shall notify the State Department of Public Health. The State Department of Public Health shall follow up all positive tests with the attending physician who notified the department thereof and with the parents of the newborn child when such notification was made by a person other than a physician, and, when confirmed, the services and facilities of the said State Department of Public Health, and those of other state boards, departments and agencies cooperating with the Department of Public Health in carrying out the program shall be made available to the extent needed by the family and physician. The State Department of Public Health and the other state departments and agencies cooperating with it shall, in cooperation with the attending physician, provide for the continued medical care, dietary and other related needs of such children, where necessary or desirable.

B.   In addition to the test prescribed by Subsection A hereof, there shall be administered to a newborn child a test for meniscocytosis, commonly known as sickle cell anemia; provided, however, that no test shall be given to any child whose parents object thereto. The attending physician, or the person attending a newborn child who was not attended by a physician, shall cause such child to be subject to such test. If the test is positive the attending physician or person shall notify the State Department of Public Health. The department shall follow up all positive tests with the attending physician who notified the department thereof and with the parents of the newborn child when such notification was made by a person other than a physician, and, when confirmed, shall inform the physician and/or parents of the services and facilities of the State Department of

Public Health and those of other state boards, departments and agencies cooperating with the Department of Public Health in carrying out the program and in cooperation with the attending physician shall be made available to the extent needed by the family and physician to provide for the continued medical care, dietary and other related needs of such children where necessary or desirable which are now, or may hereafter become, available for the care and treatment of meniscocytosis.

Amended by Acts 1972, No. 28, § 1.

Many statutes provide that only parents may object to testing for PKU, and only on religious grounds.

The PKU statutes, as well as the statutes related to ophthalmia neonatorum and the Louisiana statute concerning sickle cell anemia, illustrate the state's power to regulate preventive as well as corrective medicine.

Mandatory sickle cell screening laws have been passed in Massachusetts, the District of Columbia, Virginia, Maryland, New York, Illinois, Mississippi, Indiana, Kentucky, Georgia, Arizona, and Louisiana. However, through a concerted effort of those opposed to such statutes, legislation has been passed repealing mandatory screening laws in New York, Illinois, Massachusetts, Maryland, the District of Columbia, Georgia, and Virginia.

BIRTHS AND DEATHS

Birth certificates must be completed and signed by the attending physician for all live births and stillbirths. In some states licensed midwives have legal authority to sign birth certificates. In general a live birth is defined as any infant born at any age who shows, after birth, any signs of life. Signs of life include a heartbeat, respiratory activity, or cord impulse. These signs define life even if they exist only momentarily. Whenever an infant shows signs of life after birth, if that infant dies soon thereafter, both a birth certificate and a death certificate must be completed.

In the event of an abortion, sometimes seen in emergency rooms, usually neither a birth certificate nor a death certificate needs to be completed. However, it should be charted in the emergency record and signed by the attending physician. State regulations vary on the reporting of abortions; some states require the reporting of all abortions, while others require the reporting of induced abortions only.

Births out of wedlock are commonly a reportable event. States that require this reporting do so for the purpose of keeping accurate records and statistics on births within the state. The same rationale holds true for the reporting of deaths. North Dakota's reporting statute for births out of wedlock is typical:

§ 50-20-03 RESPONSIBILITY FOR REPORTING

Births out of wedlock or with congenital deformities which occur in a licensed maternity home or hospital shall be reported by the licensee of such home or hospital. All such births occurring outside of maternity homes or hospitals shall be reported by the legally qualified physician in attendance, or in the event of absence of a physician, by the registered nurse or other attendant.

The patient who is brought to the hospital emergency department dead on arrival (DOA) presents another reportable incident for the emergency room staff. In order to investigate the possibility of foul play and to determine whether an autopsy or post-mortem examination is warranted, DOAs are reported to the office of the coroner or medical examiner.

Once the emergency room physician has pronounced the patient dead and has notified the coroner or medical examiner, his or her responsibility is concluded. The emergency room physician and the rest of the emergency department staff should not do anything to alter the appearance of the corpse. Clothing and any other items accompanying the body should be saved for the coroner or medical examiner. A receipt should be obtained from the coroner's office for the clothing and other items transferred from the emergency department to that office.

CRIMINAL ACTS

Gunshot wound laws require reports where injuries are inflicted by lethal weapons or, in some cases, by unlawful acts. Some statutes even include automobile accidents within their definition of lethal weapons. The New York statute is typical:

§ 265.25 CERTAIN WOUNDS TO BE REPORTED (Penal Law)

Every case of a bullet wound, gunshot wound, powder burn or any other injury arising from or caused by the discharge of a gun or firearm, and every case of a wound which is likely to or may result in death and is actually or apparently inflicted by a knife, icepick or other sharp or pointed instrument shall be reported at once to the police authorities of the city, town or village where the person reporting is located by: (a) the physician attending or treating the case; or

(b) the manager, superintendent or other person in charge, whenever such case is treated in a hospital, sanitarium or other institution.

. . .

The connection of guns with crime makes this law a valid exercise of police power. Information provided by these reports is also useful for those making statistical studies of crime.

In addition to those subjects specified by statute as reportable, emergency room personnel may have a moral or legal duty to report to the police such acts as attempted suicide, assault, rape, or the unlawful dispensing or taking of narcotic drugs. Much of this information may be learned while caring for patients and would ordinarily be privileged communication. Therefore, care must be taken that only the police are given such information. When it comes to notifying the police, emergency room policies should clearly delineate what is reportable and how the report is to be made. The policies should also clearly indicate who is responsible for making the report.

In addition to the reportable incidents already described, emergency room policies should provide for the reporting of animal bites as a precaution against rabies, suspected self-inflicted injuries, drug overdoses or poisonings with an intent to commit suicide, suspected criminal abortions, as well as unsuspected food poisoning involving a commercial vendor (to preclude further injuries to customers). If the emergency department is a subdivision of a hospital located close to an armed forces base, the policies should address the situations in which armed forces police are to be notified in addition to civilian authorities.

The emergency room policies should also include guidelines for release of information to the press regarding police cases. The policies should specify who is authorized to speak to the press as the representative of the hospital emergency department. The policies should also detail how much information is to be released, whether reporters will be allowed to interview patients, how much information will be released to the press before the next of kin have been properly notified, and how much information will be released without the patient's consent. Clearly, in all of this, protection of the patient should be paramount, and the policies should include a statement to that effect.

ABUSED CHILDREN

Every society wishes the best possible environment for its members. Government acts as an agent of society in protecting its people through health statutes and regulations. Only through reliable observations and reports can proper measures be instituted to safeguard the environment of the society. Therefore, professionals in emergency health service play a very important role. Because health professionals are in a position to observe and gather information about parental neglect and abuse and mistreatment of children in general, every health professional has an obligation to report this information to the appropriate authority so that corrective measures can be taken.

Health statutes requiring that certain information regarding mistreatment and neglect of children be reported to government officials are of prime importance to emergency room staff because such cases are seen with some frequency in this setting. Although most statutory reporting requirements do not contain an express immunity from suit for disclosure, many do. The person making the report under statutory command will, as a general rule, be protected by the doctrine of privilege. There was a time when health practitioners may have had good reason to avoid reporting their suspicions about injured children. Anyone who made a report of child abuse to the proper authorities could have been sued by the child's parents on the basis that the report constituted a defamation of the parents' character or an invasion of their privacy. Health practitioners could also have been liable for money damages if their suspicions were proved wrong. Today, however, since all of the states and the District of Columbia have enacted laws to protect abused children, most statutes protect the persons required to report cases of child abuse.

Reporting statutes are the legal means by which the state regulates the health, welfare, and safety of its citizens—including children—through the exercise of the state's general police power. Although some of these reporting laws are permissive, others are mandatory. The permissive statutes allow for the discretion of the reporter in determining whether or not to report. The mandatory reporting laws require reporting by certain classes of professionals who are likely to observe and discover cases of child abuse; these statutes provide for statutory penalties of fine or imprisonment for not reporting.

Over the past decade, reporting of suspected cases of child abuse has been increasing, with some state officials being overwhelmed by the number of reported cases. There is a divergence of opinion over whether child abuse is more common now than in the past or whether we are simply seeing more of it reported.

The physically abused or neglected child is a medical, social, and legal problem. It is often difficult to determine whether a child has been abused, because it is often impossible to ascertain whether the child was injured intentionally or accidentally. In some cases—as with injuries to a very young infant or a history of repeated injuries—the determination is easier to make. Even the legal definition of a child varies. In one state a 12-year-old is an adult in the eyes of the law; in another state an 18-year-old is legally still a child. To compound the confusion, some state laws apply to minors but do not define "a minor"; others use the word "child" without further definition.

The various laws differ in their definition of an abused child. Generally, an abused child is one who has had serious physical injury inflicted by other than accidental means. The injuries may have been inflicted by a parent or by any other person responsible for the child's care. Some states extend the definition to include a child suffering from starvation. Other states include moral neglect in their definition of abuse. For example, Arizona mentions immoral associations; Idaho includes endangering the child's morals; Mississippi describes being found in a disreputable place or associating with vagrant, vicious, or immoral persons as a form of moral neglect. In a few states sexual abuse is also enumerated as an element of neglect.

Any report of child abuse must be made with a good faith belief that the facts reported are true. What "good faith" means is left ultimately to a court decision. But when a health practitioner's evaluation establishes reasonable cause to believe a child's injuries were not accidental, making the report will not result in liability. All abused child statutes provide protection from civil suit for anyone making or participating in a good faith report. Most states also provide immunity from criminal liability. In states that do not provide such immunity, it is extremely unlikely that anyone making a good faith report would be subject to criminal liability.

Laws governing the reporting of child abuse specify the nature and content of the report. Almost all the laws require that when a person covered by statute is attending a child as a staff member of a hospital or similar institution, and child abuse is suspected, the staff member must notify the person in charge of the institution, who in turn makes the necessary report. Typical statutes provide that an oral report be made immediately, followed as soon as possible by a written report. Most states require that the report contain the following information: the name and address of the child, the persons responsible for the child's care, the child's age, the nature and extent of the child's injuries (including any evidence of previous injuries), and any other information that might be helpful in establishing the cause of the injuries and the identity of the perpetrator.

As mentioned earlier in this chapter, reporting laws can be ignored only at the hospital's peril. In *Landeros* v. *Flood,* 131 Cal. Rptr. 69, 551 P. 2d 389 (1976), the California Supreme Court held a hospital liable for later injuries suffered by an abused child whom it improperly released to the care of the parents. Suit was brought by an infant child, through her guardian ad litem, charging both the hospital and the physician treating her with negligence for failing to report her abuse to the police or juvenile probation department, as required by state law. The court rationale was that it was reasonably foreseeable at the time of her release that her parents were likely to resume their abuse.

A state-by-state analysis of child abuse laws follows at the end of this chapter (see Exhibit 8-1).

PROTECTIVE LAWS FOR THE ELDERLY

In addition to cases of child abuse, the staff of emergency departments are likely to see situations of elderly abuse. In the future, as the birth rate continues to decline and life expectancy continues to climb, we may well be faced with more and more cases of elderly abuse and neglect. This might be expected because of the concomitant breakdown of the extended family in this society; a growing number of elderly persons are now living alone, far away from their relatives.

During the past decade, a number of states have enacted laws dealing with protective services for adults. Some of these statutes provide for mandatory reporting by health professionals of suspected cases of abuse and neglect, and a number of these laws are specifically aimed at the elderly.

The following 12 states presently have adult protection laws: Connecticut, Florida, Georgia, Maryland, Montana, North Carolina, Oregon, South Carolina, South Dakota, Tennessee, Washington, and Wisconsin. A few other states have enacted less comprehensive laws. Virginia presently has limited protective laws that provide for the appointment of guardians, but more comprehensive legislation has been proposed. Delaware, Nebraska, and New York presently have limited protective services legislation similar to that found in Virginia. West Virginia also has legislation proposed. New Jersey has enacted legislation that is limited to protective services for the institutionalized elderly.

The purpose of these protective services statutes is to provide essential services to people who are aged, infirm, or incapable of self-care. It is not very common for the staff of emergency rooms to see these people for health care. Adult protective service laws authorize social service agencies to investigate reports of abuse and neglect and to provide needed services.

The first section of South Carolina's law outlines the typical purpose of such laws and specifies that the personal freedom of the person helped be protected:

> Section 1. Findings. The General Assembly recognizes that there are many citizens of the state who, because of the infirmities of aging, mental retardation, other developmental or like incapacities incurred at any age, are in need of protective services. Such services should to the maximum degree of feasibility, allow the individual the same rights as other citizens, and at the same time protect the individual from exploitation, neglect, abuse and degrading treatment. This act is designed to establish those services, and assure their availability to all persons when in need of them, and to place the least possible restriction on personal liberty and exercise of constitutional rights

consistent with due process and protection from abuse, exploitation and neglect.

§ 43-29-10 to 100, South Carolina Laws (1974).

Most of these laws protect all adults. The laws in Connecticut and Tennessee limit protection to persons over the age of 60. All states define the object of their statutes as persons who, for mental or physical reasons, are incapable of self-care.

Most of the state laws require reporting by persons having reasonable cause to know of incidents of abuse or neglect. South Carolina limits this requirement to "practitioners of the healing arts," which could be inferred as physicians only. Washington's law refers only to "practitioners, licensees, and employees of the state health and social service agency." This would include all nurses and physicians.

The state laws require reports to be made first to the social service authorities, who in turn are required to report to legal authorities or permit reports to be made to either social service or legal authorities.

Most of the laws that mandate reporting grant immunity from prosecution to anyone who makes a "good faith" report of abuse or neglect. The state law in Oregon appears to be the only one that has no immunity provision for those reporting in "good faith."

Penalties exist for not reporting but they are not onerous. Connecticut's law provides that "any person required to report under the provision of this section who fails to make such report shall be fined not more than five hundred dollars" Connecticut Public Act 77-613 (1977). South Carolina has a similar provision except that the maximum penalty is $500 *or* 90 days in jail. Kentucky provides that violators be fined from $25 to $200. No cases have been found wherein health professionals have been penalized for failure to report, as is true in the laws covering child abuse. However, the laws on protective services and mandatory reporting of incidents involving elderly abuse are more recent.

It is important for emergency room staff members to note that elderly persons can be just as dependent as children when they are incapacitated due to ill health, poverty, isolation, and lack of mobility. Due to the location of the individual general hospital, the emergency staff may see a great number of elderly clients or very few indeed. Those hospitals located close to senior citizen housing tracts can expect to see such clients more frequently and should be alert to the signs and symptoms of abuse and neglect.

DRUG LAWS

State and federal laws regulate the use of drugs and the reporting of such use. Therefore, one of the areas of acute importance in delivering emergency care is the control and maintenance of drug records. Because emergency room situations frequently require immediate treatment, health professionals can become so involved in each emergency that it can become difficult to keep a careful record of drugs used. Policies and procedures that govern the use of drugs in the emergency room should be formulated and adhered to strictly in every instance.

In formulating drug policies for use in the emergency room, it is essential that the staff be involved. The staff, in consultation with hospital pharmacists, should draft drug policies that are workable and in conformance with state and federal laws.

The entire stock of the hospital pharmacy is subject to government control at all levels, but perhaps the most rigidly regulated items are the various drugs. It is imperative that the hospital administrator, pharmacist, medical staff, nurses, and all employees who are authorized to deal with drugs understand the manner in which they are regulated. The hospital attorney should be prepared to aid in the interpretation of laws and regulations dealing with drugs, and he or she should keep the administrator informed of changes and revisions as they affect the hospital.

The difference between a drug, a device, and a cosmetic is more important in hospital practice than in most other areas of practice because all kinds of products are found in wide use throughout the hospital. The Food, Drug and Cosmetic Act applies to the purity, labeling, potency, safety, and effectiveness of these products in varying degrees, depending on how they are classified. Therefore, it is important to distinguish among them. The federal Food, Drug and Cosmetic Act and federal regulations promulgated under the act should be consulted. There has been considerable litigation in this area, and these decisions must be taken into account.

A number of items used in hospitals have been held to be drugs, although they might not seem to be drugs to a casual observer. These items include antibiotic sensitivity discs used in laboratory procedures to determine the inhibiting ability of various antibiotics on sample microorganisms, diagnostic preparations listed in official compendia, and certain sutures used for tying off blood vessels during surgical procedures. Whole human blood has also been held to be a drug within the meaning of the Food, Drug and Cosmetic Act, and so have the plastic bags used to store blood and other intravenous substances.

At the present time, the Food and Drug Administration has established a special office to deal specifically with devices on the market, and special attention will be given to products affecting life itself, such as pacemakers. Legislative proposals are being considered as an answer to this problem area.

The definition of "new drug" is critical in analyzing the effect of the operative provision of the Food, Drug and Cosmetic Act. The law and regulations establish an elaborate procedure for determining whether a new drug is safe and effective. As part of this procedure, the Food and Drug Administration may condition its approval to market a new drug upon specified stipulations.

Specifically, a problem may arise if a physician prescribes a new drug for a condition or in a dosage other than that indicated in the approved labeling, and a pharmacist is asked to dispense the drug and a nurse is asked to administer it. As a general rule, physicians may prescribe and pharmacists may dispense new drugs for uses or in dosages or regimens different from those set forth in a drug's approved labeling without violation of the law.

The general law of negligence governs in cases where a new drug is used in a way other than provided for in the official labeling. In applying these principles to hospital practice, it appears prudent for a pharmacist to question a physician who prescribes a drug in a manner that deviates substantially from the package insert. In really questionable cases, the pharmacist should obtain an acknowledgment and assumption of liability form from the physician. This will provide protection to the pharmacist and hospital and possibly serve as an element in the defense of any subsequent liability suit.

Requirements for labeling specifications are set forth in the Food, Drug and Cosmetic Act and in regulations pursuant to the act. These labeling and prescription requirements are of major importance to the practice of hospital pharmacy.

When the prescription drugs are ordered in writing there is no particular problem. The physician either writes a prescription or writes the order in the patient's chart (which serves as the written prescription). However, if the order is an oral order, the act states that such a prescription must be ". . . reduced promptly to writing and filed by the pharmacist. . . ." Refills for such drugs must be treated likewise. Thus it is questionable practice to phone in drug orders to personnel other than the hospital pharmacist.

Every person who owns or operates any establishment engaged in the interstate or intrastate manufacture, preparation, propagation, compounding, or processing of drugs must register his or her name, place of business, and all establishments with the Secretary of Health and Human Services. This provision includes the repackaging of the drug or otherwise changing its container, wrapper, or labeling for distribution to others who will make final the sale or distribution to the customer.

The act also stipulates other manufacturing obligations, such as the maintenance of certain records, the filing of specified reports, and periodic plant inspections.

Although certain provisions of the federal Food, Drug and Cosmetic Act specifically apply to intrastate commerce of drugs, at various times Congress has specifically provided for the applicability of state law. Accordingly, most states now have food, drug and cosmetic laws based primarily on the Uniform State Food, Drug and Cosmetic Act. State laws vary in specific details from the uniform act or the federal act. Therefore state laws must be consulted in determining whether a specific course of conduct is in compliance with all applicable laws.

The Comprehensive Drug Abuse Prevention and Control Act of 1970, commonly known as the Controlled Substances Act, was signed into law on October 27, 1970. This law replaced virtually all preexisting federal laws dealing with narcotics, depressants, stimulants, and hallucinogens. Some portions of the law directly affect hospital distribution systems. The law also deals with rehabilitation programs under community mental health programs, research in and medical treatment of drug abuse and addiction, and importation and exportation of controlled substances. The act should be consulted carefully when setting up procedures for the handling and administering of controlled substances.

Hospitals are included under the Controlled Substances Act as "practitioners," and as such must register with the government in accordance with the provisions of the act. Each registrant must take a physical inventory every two years. In maintaining inventory records, a perpetual inventory is not required. However, a separate inventory is required for each registered location and for each independent activity that is registered. In addition to inventory records, each registrant must maintain complete and accurate records of all controlled substances received and disposed of.

Controlled substances in Schedules I through IV may, for all practical purposes, be dispensed only upon the lawful order of a practitioner. In analyzing the prescription requirements set forth in the regulations, it is important to keep in mind that chart orders for inpatients are excluded from the definition of prescription. Chart orders satisfy the act's requirements for a lawful order, and separate prescriptions are not required. Outpatient dispensing, on the other hand, is not exempt from the prescription requirements.

All registrants must provide effective controls and procedures to guard against theft and diversion of controlled substances. The hospital's central storage should be under the direct control and supervision of the pharmacist. Only authorized personnel should have access to the area. When controlled substances are stored at nursing units they should be kept securely locked, and only authorized personnel should have access to these drugs.

Until the enactment of the Controlled Substances Act, most states had adopted some version of the Uniform Narcotic Drug Act. Since Congress amended the federal law, the states have been steadily repealing their narcotic and depressant-stimulant laws and replacing them with "mini" controlled substances acts.

HANDICAPPED PATIENTS

Effective June 3, 1977, Department of Health and Human Services (HHS) regulations implementing § 504 of the Rehabilitation Act of 1973 require all health care institutions employing 15 or more persons and receiving HHS financial assistance (either in the form of Medicaid or Medicare funds or from federal grants, contracts, or construction funds) to take positive steps to assure handicapped persons equal access to patient services. The regulations, 42 F.R. 22675, also forbid hospitals to deny or limit health or social services to handicapped persons. These regulations apply to emergency health services.

For purposes of the Rehabilitation Act, a handicapped individual has been defined as either a person who has a physical or mental impairment that substantially limits one or more major life activities, or a person who has a history of such a condition or is regarded by others as having such a condition. The definition is sufficiently broad to include persons with such diseases and conditions as orthopedic, visual, speech and hearing impairments, as well as cerebral palsy, epilepsy, multiple sclerosis, cancer, heart disease, mental retardation, and emotional illness. The regulations expressly include persons suffering from alcohol or drug addiction as handicapped individuals.

By September 3, 1977, affected institutions were required to have taken appropriate steps to notify handicapped persons (including those with impaired hearing and vision) that their facilities did not discriminate on the basis of handicap in admission, treatment, or access to programs and activities. Suggested methods of notification included posting of notices, publication of notices in newspapers and magazines, or distribution of written material that communicates this assurance. In addition, affected institutions were required to adopt grievance procedures to handle discrimination complaints. The procedures must comply with appropriate due process standards.

By June 3, 1978, health care institutions, in conjunction with handicapped persons or their representative organizations, were required to evaluate their programs and policies to determine compliance with the federal regulations. They were further required to consult with handicapped persons on ways to modify noncomplying policies or procedures and on ways to remedy the effects of past discrimination. In addition, institutions must, for at least three years, maintain on file and make available for public inspection, records that identify the persons consulted and the procedures and policies examined, list the problems identified, and describe the proposed modifications or remedial steps. However, the regulations require no goals or timetables for remedial action.

The HHS regulations require that institutions offering emergency services take positive steps to facilitate communication with hearing-impaired persons, by such means as on-call interpreters or the use of written communications. Materials that constitute either a waiver of a patient's rights or a consent to certain procedures should also be produced in a way that effectively advises the handicapped of their rights. For example, in the case of blind patients, explanations should be written in Braille. Auxiliary aid for persons with impaired sensory, manual, or speaking skills must also be provided.

Although hospitals are not required to accept all alcohol and drug addiction patients, they cannot deny treatment solely because of a patient's status as an alcoholic or a drug abuser. Consequently, a cancer hospital cannot reject a cancer patient simply because the patient is an alcoholic; however, institutions may continue to refer patients whose primary illness is alcohol or drug abuse to more appropriate treatment facilities.

In order to protect against possible liability for not reporting incidents which are reportable, it is essential that the hospital make documentation. Forms used for reporting should be filled out in duplicate; one copy should be mailed to the appropriate public official, and one should be put into the patient's record.

HOSPITAL RECORDS

Various state and federal regulations and laws govern hospital records. Some states detail the information to be recorded; other states specify which broad areas of information concerning the patient's treatment must be included; some states simply declare that the medical record shall be adequate, accurate, or complete. State hospital licensure rules and regulations may also provide requirements and standards for the maintenance, handling, signing, filing, and retention of hospital records.

Federal regulations under Medicare and Medicaid, Condition of Participation—Emergency Service or Department, 20 C.F.R. §405.1033, provide for the following:

> (d) Standard; medical records. Adequate medical records on every patient are kept. The factors explaining the standard are as follows:
> (I)   The emergency room record contains:
> (i)   Patient identification.

(ii)   History of disease or injury.
(iii) Physical findings.
(iv)   Laboratory and X-ray reports, if any.
(v)   Diagnosis.
(vi)   Record of treatment.
(vii) Disposition of the case.
(viii) Signature of a physician.
(2)   Medical reports for patients treated in the emergency service are organized by a medical record librarian or her equivalent.
(3)   Where appropriate, medical records of emergency services are integrated with those of the inpatient and outpatient services.
(4)   A proper method of filing records is maintained.
(5)   At a minimum, emergency service medical records are kept for as long a time as required in a given State's statute of limitations.

In addition to specific requirements, all licensing regulations stipulate that all records must be accurate and complete. Furthermore, the Joint Commission on Accreditation of Hospitals (JCAH) and several licensing regulations require the prompt completion of records after the discharge of patients. JCAH has published Standard V on emergency services and recordkeeping: "A medical record shall be kept for every patient receiving emergency services; it shall become an official hospital record." JCAH then stipulates the minimum of what must be included in the record. In comparing the JCAH standard to the Medicare regulations, one sees a great deal of similarity in the requirements. JCAH requires:

(1)   adequate patient identification and consent;
(2)   information about the time of the patient's arrival, and by whom transported;
(3)   pertinent history of the injury or illness, including details relative to first aid or emergency care given to the patient prior to his arrival at the hospital;
(4)   vital signs;
(5)   names of attending physicians and nurses;
(6)   diagnosis and treatment given; and
(7)   final disposition, including instruction given to the patient and/ or his family relative to necessary follow-up.

In *Board of Trustees of Memorial Hospital* v. *Pratt,* 72 Wyo. 120, 262 P. 2d 682 (1953), persistent failure to conform to a medical staff rule requiring the physician to complete records promptly was held to provide a basis for suspending a staff member.

The following case shows it is essential that emergency room internal policies and procedures address the completion of hospital records by emergency room personnel. These policies should be followed scrupulously. Penalties for violators should be written into the policies and enforced when necessary.

In *Louisville General Hospital* v. *Hellmann,* 500 S.W. 2d 790 (1973), the facts revealed that a Mr. Bratcher was admitted to the defendant hospital for treatment of a head injury. He remained in the hospital for approximately two-and-one-half weeks before his death. His widow sued the hospital, claiming negligent care.

The emergency room record contained only two entries in regard to medical care the decedent had received in the emergency room between the hours of 8 p.m. and 6 a.m. on the day of admission. The physician testified that he had monitored the decedent's vital signs every 30 minutes during the time he was in the emergency room. The doctor stated that the failure to record each examination was the normal accepted procedure employed at the hospital.

In view of the doctor's testimony, the plaintiff moved that the trial court enter an order directing the hospital to produce for inspection and copying all emergency room records compiled and prepared in the ordinary course of business of the hospital for each of the 30 days immediately preceding and including April 2, 1968, the date the decedent had been admitted. This order was duly entered by the court.

The defendant hospital moved that this order be set aside, and in support filed the affidavit of Edith Frey, the Director of Medical Records, which stated that it was physically impossible to produce such records as they were filed by patient number, not by month, and that there were approximately 5,000 records involved in that 30-day period.

The court overruled this motion. The defendant hospital filed a petition for writ of prohibition. The appellate court stated that it appeared that the order would place an undue burden on the hospital, which was not commensurate with the results that might be obtained. Therefore, the trial court's order was modified to provide that the examination of the emergency room records was to be confined to no more than 100 of such records selected at random. Any personal information which might identify the patient was to be concealed.

The modified court order demonstrates the willingness of the court to look for a pattern of recording treatment in the emergency room of the defendant hospital and emphasizes the importance of hospital records in court cases.

Appendix 8A*

State by State Summary of Child Abuse Laws

Source: Cazalas, *Nursing and the Law,* 3rd ed., Appendix E (Germantown, Md.: Aspen Systems Corp., 1978).

State	Citation	Applies To
Alabama	Ala. Code Tit. 26, Section 26-14-1 (1975)	Hospitals, clinics, sanitariums, doctors, physicians, surgeons, medical examiners, coroners, dentists, osteopaths, optometrists, chiropractors, podiatrists, nurses, school teachers and officials, peace officers, law enforcement officials, pharmacists, social workers, day care workers or employees, mental health professionals, any other person called on to render aid or medical assistance to any child, or any person.
Alaska	Alaska Stat. Sections 47.17.010 to 47.17.070 (1971)	Practitioner of healing arts, school teachers, social workers, peace officers and officers of the division of corrections, administrative officers of institutions, or any other person.
Arizona	Ariz. Rev. Stat. Ann. Section 13-842.01 (1976)	Physician, hospital, intern, resident, surgeon, dentist, osteopath, chiropractor, podiatrist, medical examiner, nurse, psychologist, school personnel, social worker, peace officer, or any other person responsible for the care of children.
Arkansas	Ark. Stat. Ann. Sections 42.807-42-818 (1975)	Physician, surgeon, coroner, dentist, osteopath, resident, intern, registered nurse, hospital personnel (engaged in admission, examination, care, or treatment), teacher, school official, social service worker, day care center worker, or any other child or foster care worker, mental health professional, peace officer, law enforcement official, and any other person.
California	Cal. Penal Code Sections 11161.5 to 11161.7	Physician, surgeon, dentist, resident, intern, podiatrist, chiropractor, marriage, family or child counselor, psychologist, religious practitioner, registered nurse employed by public health agency, school or school district, superintendent or supervisor of child welfare, certified pupil personnel employee of public or private school system, principal or teacher, licensed day care worker, administrator of summary day camp or child care center, social worker, peace officer, probation officer.

Age Limit	Report To	Immunity Provision	Physician-Patient Privilege Eliminated	Penalty
18	Duly constituted authority— Chief of Police, Sheriff, Dept. of Pensions & Security or its designee but not an agency involved in the acts or omissions of reported child abuse or neglect.	Yes	Yes	Misdemeanor. Sentence 6 mos or $500.00
16	Department of Health and Welfare, peace officer.	Yes	Yes	
18	Municipal or county peace officer or protective services of state dept. of economic security.	Yes	Yes	Misdemeanor
18	Person in charge of institution or his designated agent who shall report. District or State Social Services, Division of the Department of Social and Rehabilitative Services.	Yes	Yes	Misdemeanor. Sentence 5 days and $100.00. Civil liability for damages proximately caused by failure to report.
18	Local police authority, juvenile probation department, county welfare department, county health department.	Yes		

State	Citation	Applies To
Colorado	Colo. Rev. Stat. Ann. Sections 19-10-101 through 19-10-115 (1975)	Physician or surgeon including physicians in training, child health associate, medical examiner or coroner, dentist, osteopath, optometrist, chiropractor, chiropodist or podiatrist, registered nurse, licensed practical nurse, hospital personnel engaged in admission, care, or treatment, Christian Science practitioner, school official or employee, social worker, worker in a family care home or child care center, mental health professional, any other person.
Connecticut	Conn. Gen. Stat. Rev. Section 17-38a (1973)	Physician, nurse, medical examiner, dentist, psychologist, school teacher, principal, guidance counselor, social worker, police officer, clergyman, coroner, osteopath, optometrist, chiropractor, podiatrist, any person paid to care for children or mental health professional.
Delaware	Del. Code Ann. Tit. 16 Sections 1001 to 1008 (Supp. 1972)	Physician, any person in healing arts, medicine, osteopathy, dentistry, intern, resident, nurse, school employee, social worker, psychologist, medical examiner or any other person.
Florida	Fla. Stat. Ann. Sections 827.01 to 827.09 (1977)	Physician, dentist, podiatrist, optometrist, intern, resident, nurse, teacher, social worker, employee of a public or private facility serving children.
Georgia	Ga. Code Ann. Sections 74-109 to 74-11 (1977)	Social worker, teacher, school administrator, child care personnel, day care personnel, law enforcement personnel, any other person.
Hawaii	Hawaii Rev. Stat. Sections 350-1 to 350-5 (1968), As Amended, (Supp. 7)	Doctor of medicine, osteopathy, dentistry, or any of the other healing arts, registered nurse, school teacher, social worker, medical examiner, and any other person.

Age Limit	Report To	Immunity Provision	Physician-Patient Privilege Eliminated	Penalty
Child	Local law enforcement agency or the county or district department of social services. Receiving agency is to report to central registry.	Yes	Yes	Class 2 petty offense. Fine $200.00. Civil liability for damages proximately caused by failure to report.
18	State Commission of Social Services or local police department.	Yes	Yes	$1,000.00 or one year.
*	Division of Social Services of Dept. of Health & Social Services.	Yes	Yes	Maximum of $100.00 and/or maximum of 15 days imprisonment.
17	Person in charge of institution, Department of Health and Rehabilitative Services.	Yes	Yes	Misdemeanor of second degree. Sentence 60 days, $500.00, or both.
18	Person in charge of institution and county health officer, and child welfare agency designated by Dept. of Human Resources and police authority.	Yes		Misdemeanor. Imprisonment less than 12 mos.
18	Person in charge of medical facility, Department of Social Services and Housing.	Yes	Yes	

* 18 or mentally retarded.

State	Citation	Applies To
Idaho	Idaho Code Section 16-1619 through 16-1629 (1976)	Physician, resident, intern, nurse, coroner, school teacher, day care personnel, social worker, any other person.
Illinois	Ill. Ann. Stat. Ch. 23 Sections 2051-2061 (1975)	Physician, hospital, surgeon, dentist, osteopath, chiropractor, podiatrist, Christian Science practitioner, coroner, school teacher, school administrator, truant officer, social worker, social services administrator, registered nurse, licensed practical nurse, director or staff assistant of a nursery school or a child day care center, law enforcement officer, or field personnel of the Illinois Department of Public Aid.
Indiana	Ind. Ann. Stat. Sections 12-3-4.1-1 to 12-3-4.1-6 (1973)	Any person.
Iowa	Iowa Code Ann. Sections 235A.1 to 235A.24	Health practitioner, social worker, certified psychologist, certified school employee, employee of a licensed day care facility, member of the staff of a mental health center, peace officer, any other person.
Kansas	Kan. Stat. Ann. 38-716 to 38-756	Persons licensed to practice healing art, dentistry, optometrist, engaged in postgraduate training programs approved by the state board of healing arts, certified psychologists, Christian Science practitioners, licensed social workers, every licensed professional nurse or licensed practical nurse, teacher, school administrator or other employee of a school, chief administrative officer of a medical care facility, every person licensed by the secretary of health and environment to provide child care services or employee of the person so licensed at the place where the child care services are being provided to the child, or any law enforcement officer.
Kentucky	Ky. Rev. Stat. Ann. Sec. 199.335 1964 As Amended 1970, 1972, 1974	Physician, osteopathic physician, nurse, teacher, school administrator, social worker, coroner, medical examiner, and any other person.

Age Limit	Report To	Immunity Provision	Physician-Patient Privilege Eliminated	Penalty
18	Law enforcement agency, person in charge of the institution or designee. Law enforcement report to Department of Health and Welfare.	Yes	Yes	
Child	Dept. of Child & Family Services, local law enforcement agency.	Yes	Yes	None
Child	County department of public welfare, law enforcement agency.	Yes	Yes	Misdemeanor. Sentence 30 days, $100.00, or both.
18	Dept. of Social Services, law enforcement agency.	Yes	Yes	Misdemeanor. $100.00 or 10 days. Civil liability for damages proximately caused by failure to report.
Child	District court of county in which such examination or attendance is made, treatment is given, school is located or such abuse or neglect is extant or to the department of social and rehabilitation services.	Yes	Yes	Misdemeanor
18	Person in charge of institution, Department of Human Resources.	Yes	Yes	

State	Citation	Applies To
Louisiana	La. R.S. 14:403 (1964) As Amended 1970, 1974, 1975, and 1977	Any person, physicians, interns, residents, nurses, hospital staff members, teachers, social workers, other persons or agencies having responsibility for care of children.
Maine	Me. Rev. Stat. Ann. Tit. 22 Sections 3853-3860 (1975) As Amended 1977	Any medical physician, resident, intern, medical examiner, dentist, osteopathic physician, chiropractor, podiatrist, registered or licensed practical nurse, Christian Science practitioner, teacher, school offical, social worker, homemaker, home health aide, medical or social service worker for families and children, psychologist, child care personnel, mental health professional or law enforcement official.
Maryland	Md. Ann. Code Art. 27, Sec. 35A- (1977)	Every health practitioner, educator, social worker, law enforcement officer who contacts, examines, attends, or treats a child.
Massachusetts	Mass. Ann. c. 119 Section 51A (1973) As Amended 1975 and 1977	Physician, medical intern, medical examiner, dentist, nurse, public or private, school teacher, educational administrator, guidance or family counselor, probation officer, social worker or policeman. Any other person may report.
Michigan	Mich. Statutes Ann. Section 25.248 (1)-(Mich. Comp. Law Section 722.621) (1975)	Physician, coroner, dentist, medical examiner, nurse, audiologist, certified social worker, social worker, technician, school administrator, counselor or teacher, law enforcement officer, duly regulated child care provider.
Minnesota	Minn. Stat. Ann. Section 626.556 (1975)	Professional or his delegate engaged in practice of the healing arts, social services, hospital administration, psychological or psychiatric treatment, child care, education, or law enforcement. Any person may report.
Mississippi	Miss. Code Ann. Sections 43-24-1, 43-24-7, 43-21-11, 43-23-9, 43-23-3 (1977)	Licensed doctor of medicine, dentistry, intern, resident, registered nurse, psychologist, teacher, social worker, school principal, child care giver, minister, any law enforcement officer, and all other persons.

Age Limit	Report To	Immunity Provision	Physician-Patient Privilege Eliminated	Penalty
18	Parish child welfare unit, Parish agency responsible for protection of juveniles, local or state law enforcement agency.	Yes	Yes	Misdemeanor. Sentence 6 mos. and/or $500.00.
18	Person in charge of institution, Dept. of Health & Welfare.	None	Yes	Civil violation $500.00.
18	Local Dept. of Social Services, appropriate law enforcement agency.	Yes		
18	Person in charge of institution, Dept. of Public Welfare, attorney for county and medical examiner if death occurs.	Yes	Yes	Maximum fine $1,000.00.
18	Dept. of Social Services, person in charge of institution.	Yes	Yes	Civil liability for damages proximately caused by failure to report.
Child	Local welfare agency, police department; deaths to medical examiner or coroner who will notify the local welfare agency or police department.	Yes	Yes	Misdemeanor
18	County Welfare Department which will thereafter make a referral to the person designated by the judge of the county youth court or family court.	Yes	Yes	

State	Citation	Applies To
Missouri	Mo. Ann. Stat. Sections 210.110 to 210.165 (1975)	Physician, medical examiner, coroner, dentist, chiropractor, optometrist, podiatrist, resident, intern, nurse, hospital and clinic personnel, health practitioner, psychologist, mental health professional, social worker, day care center worker or other child care worker, juvenile officer, probation or parole officer, teacher, principal or other school official, minister, Christian Science practitioner, peace officer, law enforcement official, other person with responsibility for the care of children. Any other person may report.
Montana	Mont. Rev. Code Ann. Sections 10-1300 to 10-1322 (1974) As Amended (1977)	Physician, nurse, teacher, social worker, attorney, law enforcement officer, any other person.
Nebraska	Neb. Rev. Stat. Supp. Sections 28-1501 to 28-1508 (1975)	Physician, medical institution, nurse, school employee, social worker, any other person.
Nevada	Nevada Rev. Stat. Sections 200.501 thru 200.508	Physician, dentist, chiropractor, optometrist, resident and intern licensed in Nevada, Superintendent, manager or other person in charge of a hospital or similar institution, professional or practical nurse, physician assistant, psychologist and emergency medical technician, ambulance licensed or certified to practice in Nevada, attorney, social worker, school authority, teacher, every person who maintains or is employed by a licensed child care facility or children's camp.
New Hampshire	New Hampshire Rev. Stat. Ann. Sections 169.37 to 169.45 (1975) As Amended 1975	Physician, surgeon, county medical referee, psychiatrist, resident, intern, dentist, osteopath, optometrist, chiropractor, psychologist, therapist, registered nurse, hospital personnel, Christian Science practitioner, teacher, school official, school nurse, school counselor, social worker, day care worker, any other child or foster care worker, law enforcement official, priest, minister, or rabbi or any other person.

Age Limit	Report To	Immunity Provision	Physician-Patient Privilege Eliminated	Penalty
18	Person in charge of institution, Missouri Division of Family Service, death to medical examiner or coroner who will report to the police, peace officer, prosecuting juvenile officer, Missouri Division of Family Services.	Yes	Yes	Misdemeanor. $1,000 and/or one year.
18	Dept. of Social & Rehabilitation Services, local affiliate, county attorney where child resides.	No	Yes	None
*	Dept. of Public Welfare, Police Department, town marshall, Office of Sheriff.			
18	Local office of Welfare Division of Dept. of Human Resources, any county agency authorized by juvenile courts to receive reports, any police dept. or Sheriff's office.	Yes	Yes	Gross misdemeanor. 1 to 20 years if substantial bodily harm occurs. (Could interpret to cover failure to report.)
18	Bureau of Child & Family Services, Division of Welfare, Dept. of Health & Welfare.	Yes	Yes	Misdemeanor

---

* Minor child 18 or incompetent or disabled persons or 6 years old or under left unattended in a motor vehicle.

State	Citation	Applies To
New Jersey	New Jersey Rev. Stat. Ann. Sections 9:6-8.1 to 9:6-8.7 (1974)	Any person.
New Mexico	N.M. Stat. Ann. Sections 13-14-14.1 to 13-14-14.2 (1973)	Physician, resident, intern, law enforcement officer, registered nurse, visiting nurse, school teacher, social worker, any other person.
New York	N.Y. Soc. Service Law Sections 411 to 428 (1973)	Physician, surgeon, medical examiner, coroner, dentist, osteopath, optometrist, resident, intern, registered nurse, Christian Science practitioner, hospital personnel, social services worker, school official, day care center director, peace officer, mental health professional, and any other person.
North Carolina	N.C. Cent. Stat. Sections 110-117 to 110-119 (1977)	Physician or administrator of a hospital, clinic or other medical facility to which children are brought.
North Dakota	N.D. Cent. Code Sections 50-25.1-01 to 50-25.1-14 (1975) As Amended, 1977	Physician, nurse, dentist, optometrist, medical examiner or coroner, any other medical or mental health professional, school teacher or administrator, school counselor, social worker, day care center or any other child care worker, police, law enforcement officer, and any other person.
Ohio	Ohio Rev. Code Ann. Section 2151-42.1 (1977)	Attorney, physician, intern, resident, dentist, podiatrist, practitioner of a limited branch of medicine or surgery as defined in section 4731.15 of the Revised Code, registered or licensed practical nurse, visiting nurse, or other health care professional, licensed psychologist, speech pathologist or audiologist, coroner, administrator or employee of a child day-care center, or administrator or employee of a certified child care agency or other public or private children services agency, school teacher, or school authority, social worker, or person rendering spiritual treatment through prayer in accordance with the tenets of a well recognized religion.

Age Limit	Report To	Immunity Provision	Physician- Patient Privilege Eliminated	Penalty
18	Bureau of Child Services, Division of Youth and Family Services.	Yes		Misdemeanor. (Disorderly person).
18	County Social Services Office of the Health & Social Services Dept. in the county of child's residence or Probation Services Office in Judicial District of child's residence.	Yes	Yes	Misdemeanor. $25.00 minimum and $100.00 maximum.
*	Statewide Central Register of Child Abuse and Maltreatment Local Child Protective Service, person in charge of institution.	Yes	Yes	Class A Misdemeanor. Civil liability for damages proximately caused by failure to report.
18	Director of Social Services of county where child resides, parents, other caretakers.			
18	Division of Community Services of the Social Service Board of North Dakota.	Yes	Yes	Class B Misdemeanor.
18	Person in charge of institution, Children Services Board or County Dept. of Welfare exercising the children services function or municipal or county police officer in county of child's residence or where abuse or neglect occurred.	Yes		

* Abused 16, maltreated 18

State	Citation	Applies To
Oklahoma	Okla. Stat. Ann. Tit. 21 Sections 845-848 1965, As Amended 1977	Physician, surgeon, dentist, osteopathic physicians, residents, interns, every other person.
Oregon	Ore. Rev. Stat. Sections 418.740 to 418.775 (1975)	Public or private official, physician, intern, resident, dentist, school employee, licensed practical or registered nurse, employee of Dept. of Human Resources, County Health Dept., Community Mental Health Program, County juvenile dept, licensed child caring agency, peace officer, psychologist, clergyman, social worker, optometrist, chiropractor, certified provider of day care or foster care, attorney, law enforcement agency, police department, sheriff's office, county juvenile department.
Pennsyl-vania	Pa. Stat. Ann. Tit. 11 Sections 2201 to 2224 (1975)	Any person who in the course of their employment, occupation, or practice of their profession contacts children, licensed physician, medical examiner, coroner, dentist, osteopath, optometrist, chiropractor, podiatrist, intern, registered nurse, licensed practical nurse, hospital personnel engaged in the admission, examination, care or treatment of persons, a Christian Science practitioner, school administrator, school teacher, school nurse, social services worker, day care center worker or any other child care or foster care worker, mental health professional, peace officer or law enforcement official.
Rhode Island	R.I. Gen. Laws Ann. Sections 40-11-1 to 40-11-17 (1976)	Physicians, and any person.
South Carolina	S.C. Code Ann. Sections 20-9-10 to 20-9-70 (1962) As Amended 1972, 1974, 1976	Practitioners of healing arts, resident, intern, registered nurse, visiting nurse, school teacher, social worker, any other person.
South Dakota	S.D. Compiled. Laws Ann. Sections 26-10-11, 26-10-15 (1964) As Amended 1973, 1976	Physician, surgeon, dentist, doctor of osteopathy, chiropractor, optometrist, podiatrist, psychologist, social worker, hospital intern or resident, law enforcement officer, teacher, school counselor, school official, nurse, or coroner.

Age Limit	Report To	Immunity Provision	Physician-Patient Privilege Eliminated	Penalty
18	County office of the Dept. of Institutions, Social & Rehabilitative Services where injury occurred.	Yes	Yes	Misdemeanor
18	Local office of Children's Services Division, law enforcement agency.	Yes	No	Fine $250.00.
18	Person in charge of institution or agency, Dept. of Public Welfare of the Commonwealth of Pennsylvania.	Yes	Yes	First failure to report is a summary offense, subsequent failure to report is a misdemeanor of the third degree.
18	Director of Social & Rehabilitative Services, law enforcement agency.	Yes	Yes	
18	County Dept. of Social Services, County Sheriff's office, Chief County law enforcement officer.	Yes	Yes	Misdemeanor. Sentence: 6 mos. and/or $500.00.
18	Person in charge of institution.	Yes	Yes	Class I misdemeanor.

State	Citation	Applies To
Tennessee	Tenn. Code Ann. Sections 37-1201, 37-1212 (1973) As Amended 1975	Any person.
Texas	Tex. Family Code Ann. Sections 34.01 to 34.06 (1975)	Any person.
Utah	Utah Code Ann. Sections 55-16-1 to 55-16-6 (1975)	Any person.
Vermont	Vt. Stat. Ann. Sections 1351 to 1355 (1974) As Amended 1975, 1976 and 1977	Physician, surgeon, osteopath, chiropractor or physician assistant licensed or registered, resident physician, intern, or any hospital administrator, psychologist, school teacher, day care worker, school principal, school guidance counselor, mental health professional, social worker, probation officer, clergyman or any other person.
Virginia	Va. Code Ann. Sections 63.1-248.1 to 63.1-248.17 (1975)	Persons licensed to practice healing arts, residents, interns, nurses, social workers, probation officers, teachers, persons employed in a public or private school, kindergarten or nursery, persons providing child care for pay on a regular basis, Christian Science practitioner, mental health professional, law enforcement officer. Any person may report.
Washington	Wash. Rev. Code Ann. Sections 26.44.010 to 26.44.900 (1975)	Practitioner, professional school personnel, nurse, social worker, psychologist, pharmacist, employee of social or health services. Any person may report.
Wisconsin	Wis. Stat. Ann. Section 48.981 (1974)	Physician, surgeon, nurse, hospital administrator, dentist, social worker, school administrator.

Age Limit	Report To	Immunity Provision	Physician-Patient Privilege Eliminated	Penalty
*	Judge with juvenile jurisdiction Tennessee Dept. of Human Resources, Office of Sheriff, law enforcement official where child resides, person in charge of institution.	Yes	Yes	Misdemeanor. $50.00 and/or 3 months.
**	State Dept. of Public Welfare, Agency designated by court to protect children, local or state law enforcement.	Yes	Yes	Class B Misdemeanor.
18	Local city police, county sheriff's office, Office of the Division of Family Services, person in charge of institution.	Yes	Yes	Misdemeanor
***	Commissioner of Social & Rehabilitative Services.	Yes		Fine $100.00.
18	Person in charge of institution or department, Department of Welfare of the county or city where child resides or abuse or neglect occurred, juvenile and domestic relations district court if an employee of the Department of Welfare is the one suspected of abusing the child.	Yes	Yes	First failure to report $500.00. Subsequent failure to report $100.00 to $1,000.00.
†	Law enforcement agency, Department of Social & Health Services.	Yes		Misdemeanor
††	County Child Welfare Agency, sheriff, city police department.	Yes	†††	Sentence 6 months and/or $100.00.

---

  * 18, reasonably presumed to be under 18
 ** 18 who has not been married
*** Under age of majority
  † 18, any mentally retarded person
 †† 18 (Section 48.02)
††† See Section 325.21

State	Citation	Applies To
West Virginia	West Va. Code Ann. Sections 49-6A.1 to 49-6A-10 (1977)	Medical, dental, mental health professional, Christian Science practitioner, religious healer, school teacher, or other school personnel, social service worker, child care or foster care worker, peace officer, law enforcement official. Any other person may report.
Wyoming	Wyo. Stat. Ann. Sections 14-28.1 to 14-28.13 (1974)	Physician, surgeon, dentist, osteopath, chiropractor, podiatrist, intern, resident, nurse, druggist, pharmacist, laboratory technician, school teacher or administrator, social worker, any other person.
District of Columbia	D.C. Code Ann. Sections 2-161 to 2-169 (1977)	Physician, psychologist, medical examiner, dentist, chiropractor, registered nurse, licensed practical nurse, person involved in the care and treatment of patients, law enforcement officer, school official, teacher, social service worker, day care worker, and mental health professional. Any person may report.

Age Limit	Report To	Immunity Provision	Physician-Patient Privilege Eliminated	Penalty
18	Local State Department Child Protective Services Agency, report deaths to medical examiner or coroner.	Yes	Yes	Misdemeanor. Sentence 10 days and/or $100.00.
19	Person in charge of institution, Department of Health & Social Services, Division of Public Assistance & Social Services.	Yes	Yes	
18	Person in charge of institution, Metropolitan Police Department of the District of Columbia, Child Protective Services Division of the Department of Human Resources.	Yes	Yes	Sentence 30 days and/or $100.00.

Chapter 9

Federal Regulations

Regulations of a government agency or department are rules relating to the subject on which a department acts. Regulations are issued by the department or agency head under some act of Congress or act of a state legislature that empowers the head of the department or agency to make regulations. Therefore, although regulations are not made by judges or legislatures, they do have the force of law.

It must be remembered that regulations specifically define areas of legislation and are written to implement the law. Thus regulations written to implement a law must not go beyond the law by including subjects outside the legislation. Problems arising from regulations that reach beyond the legislation to be implemented are frequently a source of litigation. By looking at the statute and the regulations, courts are able to reach decisions believed to be in accord with the legislative intent of the law when enacted.

The power to write and implement regulations is a delegated one. The power is delegated by the legislative body to a government agency. There are many arguments, pro and con, regarding the delegation of rule-making power to government agencies. The arguments usually address the amount of power delegated by legislature rather than the delegation itself. Opponents of delegation believe that *elected* representatives of the people should not delegate rule-making power to *appointed* agency and department heads. Proponents counter by explaining that without delegation, many enacted statutes would never be implemented at all.

Realistically, if a legislature refused to delegate its power, there would be two alternatives: (1) to not implement the legislation; or (2) to make the legislature assume the responsibility for implementation. Neither alternative seems practical.

Regulations, focusing on many different areas, have an impact on the delivery of emergency health care. This chapter will deal with these various regulations.

CIVIL RIGHTS

Civil rights are guaranteed by the United States Constitution and additionally by acts of Congress and by state legislatures. Basically, civil rights refer to all the rights of each individual in a free society. In discussing civil rights as this issue relates to emergency care, there are several provisions important to know. The first is the Civil Rights Act of 1964, because it contains provisions relating to hospitals. The second is the Hill-Burton Act which specifies certain requirements for hospitals receiving aid under its program. The third is the Rehabilitation Act of 1973, which protects the physically and mentally handicapped from discrimination in health care. In addition to these federal provisions, some state laws deal with discriminatory admission policies in hospitals and in other health facilities and institutions.

It is clear that hospitals have a legal responsibility in the enforcement of civil rights. In its dealings with patients, visitors, and employees, a hospital is prohibited by law from making discriminatory distinctions based on race, color, religion, sex, or national origin.

Discrimination

Discriminatory practices in hospitals and other health facilities have been dealt with by Congress and the federal courts. Discrimination in the admission and treatment of patients, as well as the segregation of patients on racial grounds, is, for all practical purposes, proscribed in any hospital receiving federal financial assistance. Pursuant to Title VI of the Civil Rights Act of 1964, the guidelines of the Department of Health and Human Services (HHS) require that there be no racial discrimination practiced by any hospital or agency receiving money under any program supported by HHS. This includes all hospitals which are "providers of service" receiving federal funds under Medicare legislation.

According to the Fourteenth Amendment to the Constitution, a state cannot act so as to deny to any person equal protection under the law. If a state or a political subdivision of a state—whether through its executive, judicial, or legislative branch—acts in any way that unfairly denies to one person the right accorded to another, the amendment has been violated. The acts of the executive, judicial, and legislative branches of government encompass the acts of government agencies as well, and "state action" has been extended to include activities of nongovernment entities under certain circumstances. For example, if the state supports or authorizes an activity for the benefit of the public, it is possible that a nongovernment institution engaging in such activity may be considered to be engaged in state action and subject to the Fourteenth Amendment.

Considering the constitutional requirements together with the HHS guidelines and Title II of the Civil Rights Act of 1964 (which prohibits discrimination in restaurants and other places of public accommodation and thus may include restaurants in hospitals), it is apparent that racial discrimination is prohibited in practically all hospitals.

The Civil Rights Act of 1964 is particularly important because it provides that a hospital must treat nurses, patients, physicians, and other employees in a nondiscriminatory manner. Title VII of the Civil Rights Act of 1964 makes it illegal to deny equal job opportunities on the basis of race, color, religion, sex, or national origin; it also prohibits employees of the hospital from discriminating against patients, physicians, or fellow employees.

State Laws and Regulations

Most states have enacted laws to protect the civil rights of their citizens. Additionally, many states have amended their state constitutions to provide constitutional protection. Some of the state laws declare that life, liberty, and the pursuit of happiness should not be denied; others adhere closely to the language of federal civil rights legislation.

For example, the Massachusetts Civil Rights Act forbids discrimination in places of "public accommodation, resort or amusement" against persons who belong to any religious sect, creed, class, race, color, sex, denomination, or nationality. The statute defines the phrase "place of public accommodation, resort or amusement" to include hospitals, dispensaries, and clinics operating for profit. However, it excludes places owned or operated by any religious, racial, or denominational institution or organization, as well as any organization operated for charitable or educational purposes.

The Pennsylvania Human Relations Act is somewhat similar to the Massachusetts act in that it specifically includes dispensaries, clinics, and hospitals within its definition of public accommodation, resort, or amusement. But the Pennsylvania act does not apply to distinctly private institutions.

Missouri's act is not as specific as either the Pennsylvania law or the Massachusetts law. It does not specifically mention hospitals within its coverage. However, the phrase "places of public accommodation" would seem to include hospitals, since the definition includes all places or businesses offering services, facilities, and accommodations for the peace, comfort, health, welfare, and safety of the general public.

Some state laws still require separation of the races or other discriminatory practices in government and private institutions, including hospitals. The methods and manner of discrimination vary. Although these laws remain on the books, they are not valid. If they were attacked in the courts, they would be ruled unconstitutional.

Hospital Admission and Emergency Treatment

As discussed earlier, usually no legal problems arise when a hospital accepts a patient through formal arrangements made beforehand by the patient's physician. On the other hand, there may be legal difficulties when a hospital does not want to treat an individual who presents himself or herself for emergency care or when a hospital does not want to treat a patient recommended for admission by a physician without admitting privileges.

Statutes and hospital regulations that require a period of residency within the state as a basis for admission to a public hospital have been held unconstitutional, since such requirements deny the equal protection guaranteed by the Fourteenth Amendment.

The courts have been reluctant to depart from the traditional view that no person has a positive right to be admitted to a hospital. Generally, this reluctance has been displayed with respect to charitable and government hospitals as well as proprietary hospitals. Discrimination in admission practices on the basis of race, color, creed, sex, or national origin may constitute a violation of the laws forbidding discrimination. Yet such a provision merely forbids the use of these criteria; it does not establish positive rights to be admitted. In judicial decisions, the courts have displayed a marked tendency to adhere to the traditional view, but they have found other bases for imposing a duty on hospitals to admit persons for care under various circumstances. Thus they have established a clear mandate that hospitals must provide treatment for all patients seeking emergency care.

In *Hill* v. *Ohio County,* 468 S.W. 2d 306, cert. denied, 404 U.S. 1041 (Ky., 1972) a pregnant woman was denied admission, even though she stated that she was afraid she would deliver her baby before she could get back to her physician in another state. The original denial of admission was by a nurse working for the hospital, but two of the four members of the hospital's medical staff, when contacted, refused to authorize admission. The woman delivered at home, unattended, was rushed to another hospital for care, but was dead on arrival. The court held:

> In the instant case, the decedent was not admitted to the hospital nor was the element of critical emergency apparent. The hospital nurse acted in accordance with valid rules for admission to the facility. The uncontradicted facts demonstrate that no breach of duty by the hospital occurred.
>
> *Hill* v. *Ohio County* 468 S.W. 2d 306, 309.

Therefore, the hospital and the nurse were entitled to dismissal of the suit as a matter of law.

However, in *Wilmington General Hospital* v. *Manlove,* 54 Del. 15, 174 A. 2d 135 (1961), because it seemed apparent that the condition was an emergency, a different decision was rendered. This case concerned the refusal of a nurse on emergency duty in a charitable hospital to examine or treat an infant who had been suffering from diarrhea and high fever. The child died several days later. The court held that where a private hospital maintains an emergency unit, refusal to render service to a person in an "unmistakable emergency" may give rise to liability when such refusal causes injury. The rationale of the court was based on a finding that there existed an invitation to the patient to seek emergency care from the hospital. The case was sent back to the trial court where the plaintiff was to cite evidence showing some incompetency of the nurse or some breach of duty or negligence. The plaintiff thus had to show that the nurse should have realized there was an emergency or that it was her duty to call the intern in every case.

The distinction between these two cases is the judicial recognition that a hospital that maintains an emergency service may not refuse to give treatment without any valid reason to one who appears to, and in fact does, require emergency attention. The theory underlying this position is that during the time a person is making a fruitless attempt to obtain aid, his or her condition may be deteriorating. Thus courts apply the principle that the hospital's operation of an emergency service constitutes an invitation to those in need of aid.

In addition to the foregoing principle, there is an adjoining theory of reliance. In *Stanturf* v. *Sipes,* 447 S.W. 2d 558 (Mo., 1969), the Missouri Supreme Court reversed a summary judgment in favor of the defendant, a hospital administrator who had refused to allow a patient to be admitted because of an inability to pay a $25 admission charge. The patient won the right to a further hearing on his case by either a judge or jury. The court held that the hospital "was the only hospital in the immediate area, it maintained an emergency service, and . . . plaintiff applied for emergency treatment and was refused . . . ."

> The members of the public . . . had reason to rely on the [hospital's practice] and in this case it could be found that plaintiff's condition was caused to be worsened by the delay resulting from the futile efforts . . . to obtain treatment from the . . . [h]ospital.
> *Stanturf* v. *Sipes,* 447 S.W. 2d 558.

THE HILL-BURTON ACT OF 1946

Although the Hill-Burton Act is not customarily thought of as "planning" legislation, it did provide an initial planning carrot for those seeking federal funding under its terms. As a prerequisite to participation, each state was required to adopt a plan, based on surveys and inventories of existing facilities; according to which determinations of need could be made.

Clearly the Hill-Burton Act was primarily a federal program to provide financial assistance to public and nonprofit community hospitals for construction or modernization. It was administered through the regional HEW offices, which had project-approval authority. Each state had a Hill-Burton agency for distributing the funds and providing consulting services. To receive assistance, a proposed project had to conform to a published annual state plan for construction of hospitals and other health facilities, based on surveys and inventories. The project also had to meet established structural and program requirements. Grants did not have to be repaid if the constructed or modernized facility continued to operate as a health facility for a period of 20 years. Thus, even though Hill-Burton was not thought of as planning legislation, it did provide planning incentives both to states and to those health facilities seeking federal assistance for capital investment.

One obligation of Hill-Burton hospitals brought to light by litigation initiated in the early 1970s is the requirement that the hospital provide a reasonable volume of services to persons unable to pay. This service obligation can be met in one of three ways under HHS regulations:

1. by certifying that an amount of free care was provided equal to three percent of operating costs;
2. by certifying that the amount of free care provided was ten percent of all federal assistance, or
3. by maintaining an open door policy so that no person will be turned away for lack of money.

This free service obligation continues for 20 years after the grant.

An additional obligation—the nondiscrimination clause—has been the basis for civil rights suits beginning in the early 1960s. All portions and services of the facility are to be made available without discrimination, and no professional person may be discriminated against with respect to privileges of practice in the facility. This obligation was broadened by the Civil Rights Act of 1964, discussed previously.

The National Health Planning Act incorporates the Hill-Burton program and provides a structure for continuing it, although few funds are presently available for grants.

The specific statutory language requiring assurance by Hill-Burton hospitals of uncompensated care and community service is found in 42 United States Code §291(c):

[A]ssurance shall be received by the State from the applicant that (1) the facility or portion thereof to be constructed or modernized will be made available to all persons residing in the territorial area of the applicant; and (2) there will be made available in the facility or portion thereof to be constructed or modernized a reasonable volume of services to persons unable to pay therefor, but an exception shall be made if such a requirement is not feasible from a financial viewpoint.

In *Cook* v. *Ochsner,* 559 F. 2d 968 (5th Cir., 1977), the U.S. Court of Appeals for the Fifth Circuit faced the issue of the amount of free care that must be provided to indigent patients by a hospital receiving Hill-Burton financial assistance funds. The court rejected the claim that an HEW regulation formulating the amount of free patient care required was contrary to the Hill-Burton Act because the regulation failed to assure that the hospital provide free patient care to a state's entire indigent population.

The HEW regulation 42 C.F.R. Sec. 53.111 stated that a hospital is in "presumptive compliance" with Hill-Burton requirements if it provides free care in an amount equal to the lesser of three percent of its operating costs or ten percent of all federal assistance received. The court stated that the regulation "merely quantified or set forth in specific terms, as Congress intended, the amount of charity services which constituted a 'reasonable volume' of such services." A state must utilize its "entire arsenal of hospital services" to satisfy its statutory obligation; and, therefore, no one hospital is required to provide sufficient services to satisfy the needs of all indigents in its territorial area, the court reasoned. A hospital, it concluded, must only provide a reasonable amount of free indigent patient care.

In *Newsom* v. *Vanderbilt University,* 453 F. Supp. 401 (D.C. Tenn., 1978), a patient who was indebted to a hospital filed a class action suit against the facility claiming that it failed to fulfill its Hill-Burton obligation to provide a reasonable volume of uncompensated services. She alleged that 42 C.F.R. Sec. 53.111(f),—an HEW regulation (effective October 6, 1975) forbidding hospitals from characterizing uncollectible patient bills as satisfying their Hill-Burton obligation—was disregarded regularly by the hospital. This was true, she argued, because the hospital generally delayed determining a patient's Hill-Burton eligibility until after billing was completed. The court reasoned that since these patient costs could not therefore be termed Hill-Burton free services, it followed that the hospital had failed to provide adequate volume of such care. Accordingly, the court ordered the facility to offer increased levels of free services to compensate for this "deficit."

Next the court turned its attention to the patient's complaint that the hospital's procedure for distributing free care was arbitrary, and therefore in violation of the patient's procedural due process rights. Medical care is a "basic necessity of life," and, the court noted, there is a "need for procedural regularity in the allocation" of this precious resource. To assure that each application for assistance is accorded fair treatment, the court mandated that certain procedures—not presently adhered to by the hospital—be followed before a patient's Hill-Burton coverage could be denied. Patients, the court continued, must be "afforded meaningful notice of their potential eligibility to receive [free] care and of the written eligibility criteria upon which the hospital will base its determination. . . ." Also patients must be notified in writing of the reason for a denial and be given an opportunity to offer evidence supporting their application (*Newsom* v. *Vanderbilt University,* 453 F. Supp. at 424).

The court also addressed the issue of whether 42 C.F.R. Sec. 53.111(i)—requiring each hospital to "post notice" of its Hill-Burton obligation—satisfies due process by giving patients adequate notice of their potential eligibility for free care. Since it is unrealistic to believe that a distressed patient entering a hospital will see the posted notice, be curious enough to read it, fully comprehend its meaning, and assert his or her rights, the court concluded that the notice requirement failed to satisfy due process guarantees. In its place, the court concluded, HEW should promulgate a regulation ensuring that the notice of the facility's Hill-Burton obligation actually be read by or to the patient upon admission. Compare *Croft* v. *Edwards,* 353 So. 2d 669 (Fla. App., 1978), wherein a patient claimed, following treatment, that the hospital's Hill-Burton obligation to offer a reasonable volume of free care excused his nonpayment for services rendered. This argument was meritless, reasoned a Florida appeals court, since the patient failed to allege that the hospital had failed to fulfill its statutory free care obligation.

In *Cloud* v. *Regenstein,* No. 77-599A (N.D. Ga., April 29, 1977), a hospital that received Hill-Burton Act funds adopted a policy requiring nonemergency patients to make advance payments for most types of medical care. A group of patients sought an injunction barring implementation of that policy, asserting that prepayments were in violation of the act and its regulations, notably the requirements that a "reasonable volume of services" be provided to medical indigents and that services be provided to all members of the community on an equal access basis. They further claimed that the prepayment requirement might act to deny necessary services to those unable to tender cash in advance, thereby contravening the stated purpose of the act—to make care available to indigent patients.

The U. S. District Court refused to issue an injunction, finding the advance payment policy to be merely a collection procedure or administrative function, not within the scope of the act. The hospital had met its Hill-Burton obligations by rendering medical care to most patients at less than full cost; and, the court concluded, the act does not require that credit be extended to those same patients as well.

In *Euresti* v. *Stenner,* 458 F. 2d 1115 (1st Cir., 1972), an action was brought against the administrators, trustees, and county commissioners who operated a county hospital for a declaratory judgment that county residents who were unable to pay for hospital service, and others similarly situated, had the right to a reasonable volume of services. The lower court had dismissed the action and the plaintiffs appealed. The Court of Appeals reversed and remanded, holding that inasmuch as the statute providing for the federal grant of funds to build or modernize hospital facilities was intended to ensure that the indigent would be supplied sufficient hospital services when needed, a civil remedy could be implied for indigents to enforce the provisions without the existence of a formal contractual relationship. The court felt that, in any event, a contractual relationship did exist by virtue of a contract between operators of the hospital and the state which incorporated the federal statutory obligation. Thus the indigents had standing to maintain this action to enforce the obligation.

In its decision the appellate court pointed out that the lower court had concluded that no contractual relationship existed between the United States and those responsible for operation of the county hospital, and that, therefore, the hospital's receipt of $1.6 million in federal funds created no obligations upon it enforceable by either the United States or by the plaintiffs. The appellate court decided that its view of the Hill-Burton Act, and projects undertaken as a result of this law, led to a different conclusion. The court stated that there was no doubt that by adopting this portion of the act, Congress intended to benefit indigents in the position of the plaintiffs. By looking at congressional intent, the court concluded that Congress expressed its purpose as "to assist the several states in the carrying out of their programs . . . to furnish adequate hospital, clinic, or similar services to all their people . . ." (42 U.S.C. Sec. 291(a) as quoted in *Euresti* v. *Stenner,* 458 F. 2d 1115, 1117). An examination of the legislative history of the bill also indicated congressional concern for providing hospital services for indigents. It showed that when the bill was first referred to the Senate Committee, it did not contain the language now in question. During these hearings a medical officer for the Department of Agriculture suggested that the bill be revised to include "safeguards to ensure that hospitals will continue to carry out the purposes on which approval for their construction was based " (*Euresti* v. *Stenner,* at 1118).

Thereafter, when the bill was reported to the Senate, it contained the more specific provision of Sec. 291c. Thus the legislative history and the expressed purposes of Congress indicate that the act was passed to ensure that the indigent would be supplied with sufficient hospital services when needed. With this clear intent, no court had ever decided that the language of the act included no explicit indication that indigents were to have a right to enforce the act's provisions. The court stated that a civil remedy may be implied for those clearly within the protective realm of legislation or regulations in the public interest. The implication of such a right was not dependent on the existence of a formal contractual relationship. But the court then went on to say that even if a contractual relationship were required, it was found by the court to exist. The contract between the operators of the county hospital and the state explicitly incorporated the federal statutory obligation. In turn, the court stated, the state's obligation to provide assurance of compliance is the essential requirement for the furnishing of federal funds. In receiving federal funds, the court noted, the hospital operators obligated themselves to dispense a reasonable amount of free hospital services to those unable to pay. Having established the obligation, the court stated that it was clear that the plaintiffs had standing to enforce that obligation.

In a later case, *Saine* v. *Hospital Authority of Hall County,* 502 Fed. 2d 1033 (1st Cir., 1974), a similar suit was brought. The facts showed that the plaintiff was sent to defendant's hospital for x-rays. These x-rays were refused because she could not make an immediate payment. She brought suit in a district court claiming that she was refused medication and hospital care to which she was entitled under the provisions of the Hill-Burton Act, and that the hospital did not make available a reasonable volume of services to persons unable to pay therefor. Suit was dismissed in the lower court. However, on appeal, the court decided to follow *Euresti* v. *Stenner* and reversed.

In a series of actions against the defendant hospital and various government officials, *Corum* v. *Beth Israel Medical Center,* 359 F. Supp. 909 (2nd Cir., 1973) and 373 F. Supp. 550 and 558 (1974), plaintiffs attacked certain regulations promulgated to implement the sections of the Hill-Burton Act requiring recipients to provide a reasonable volume of services to those unable to pay. At issue were the rulings affecting the kinds of services a recipient hospital has to provide the poor, the presumptive compliance guidelines, the 20-year limitation on the recipient's obligation to provide services, and the rule allowing a funded facility to postpone determination of a person's ability to pay until after a bill has been sent and remains unpaid. The plaintiffs argued that all these regulations were contrary to the legislative intent of Congress in that they unduly restricted the access of the poor to the federally funded facilities.

The court found that the act required recipients to provide such services in such portion or portions of its facility as would constitute a reasonable volume in light of community needs and the amount of the grant. It also upheld the compliance guideline of uncompensated services at a level not less than the lesser of three percent of operating costs or ten percent of Hill-Burton funds or a certification that the facility would not exclude anyone for inability to pay. It upheld the 20-year limitation on the obligation of the recipient of funds to provide services to those unable to pay. The court struck down the regulation [42 C.F.R. § 553, 111 (f) (1)] allowing a facility to postpone determination of inability to pay until after the bill has been sent and remains unpaid, holding that the determination of inability to pay must be made before services are rendered.

Thus, the kinds of services a Hill-Burton hospital will provide to fulfill its obligation to those unable to pay must be determined in light of several factors. Simply opening the emergency room to them, for example, may not be adequate. Additionally, a quick and efficient system of determining financial need must be implemented for those portions of the facility providing the free or reduced-rate service.

In another suit based on the Hill-Burton Act, the issue was slightly different. In *John T. Mather Memorial Hospital, Etc.* v. *Marco,* 97 Misc. 2d 953, 413 N.Y.S. 2d 88 (1979), the issue revolved around a collection suit a hospital brought against a former patient who had not paid the balance she owed the hospital for medical services. In defense, Nancy Della Marco argued that the hospital had failed to uphold its obligation, as a recipient of Hill-Burton funds, to provide her with free treatment. She argued that she was unable to pay for the treatment and therefore was entitled to free hospital treatment.

The hospital agreed that it had an obligation under the Hill-Burton Act to provide a reasonable volume of service below cost or without charge, but it questioned whether the defendant could refuse to pay for services and base her defense on the fact that the hospital was not in compliance with the Hill-Burton Act. The court held that the defendant could not use the Hill-Burton violations as a defense. The court stated:

> It is clear that although an individual has standing to bring an action to compel compliance with the Hill-Burton Act, he must exhaust the available administrative remedies. In the case presently before the court there is no indication that the defendant has even pursued an administrative remedy. Yet the defendant would have the court circumvent the available administrative remedies [complaint filed with Secretary of HEW, with dismissal by Secretary, or Attorney General not brought a civil action for compliance with assurance to provide a reasonable volume of below-cost services within six months after

the date on which the complaint was filed with the Secretary, 42 U.S.C. § 300 p-2(c)] and make a finding that the plaintiff hospital has violated the Hill-Burton Act. This court is not prepared to take on such an onerous burden.

John T. Mather Memorial Hospital, Etc. v. *Marco,*
413 N.Y.S. 2d 88, 89.

Citing from an earlier case on the same issue, the court stated:

To allow such a defense would introduce into every hospital collection case, in addition to the usual issues, such as the rendition of services in question, the reasonableness of the charges, the liability of the defendant for the particular services rendered, such varied and collateral issues as the efforts of the hospital to provide a reasonable volume of below cost or free medical services, the economic conditions of the area served by the hospital, contributions from charitable corporations, the budget of the hospital, the determination of the class to be benefited by Hill-Burton funds, and whether the defendant as a member of the "working poor" was qualified for inclusion at the time of the rendition of services. Also, the defendant would be required to show the failure of the hospital on any given date to provide a sufficient percentage of care mandated by the (Hill-Burton) act. It cannot reasonably be said that the act ever implied the creation of such a right in an individual defendant as a defense in an action similar to that involved herein.

Yale-New Haven Hospital v. Matthews, 32 Conn. Sup. 539, 343 A.
2d 661, 664 (1974), cert. denied, 423, U.S. 1024, 96 S. Ct. 467,
46 L. Ed. 2d 398.

This case outlines the parameters around the hospital's Hill-Burton obligations by limiting a defendant in a debt collection case to issues and arguments directly connected to the debt. A patient wishing to bring a case charging that a hospital is not complying with the provision that a sufficient percentage of care be given free of charge, must follow the administrative procedure prescribed by law.

THE REHABILITATION ACT OF 1973

Passage of the Rehabilitation Act by Congress in 1973 gave the handicapped certain rights. Specifically, it protects the physically and mentally handicapped from discrimination in education, employment, transportation, housing, and health care.

This law applies to recipients of federal funds, including hospitals that receive Medicare funds under Title XVIII of the Social Security Act, or Medicaid funds under Title XIX of the Social Security Act. The specific language of the law in 29 U.S. Code 794 states:

> No otherwise qualified handicapped individual in the United States . . . shall, solely by reason of his handicap, be excluded from the participation in, be denied the benefits of, or be subjected to discrimination under any program or activity receiving Federal financial assistance.

Compliance with the law requires that health care services be provided in a nondiscriminatory way. The handicapped person must have access to any service available to a nonhandicapped person. This means that a health care facility may not deny admission for services on the basis of a handicap. For example, a hospital may not deny admission to an alcoholic or a drug addict on the basis of the drug or alcohol problem—if the person presents a medical problem. Similarly, a psychiatric clinic may not deny services on the basis that the applicant is blind.

The law requires that a hospital that receives federal dollars from Medicare and Medicaid reimbursements must be functional and accessible to physically handicapped patients, personnel, and visitors.

The requirements, under the law, are more stringent for larger facilities than they are for small ones. Institutions and other deliverers of service that have more than 15 persons associated with their operation must be accessible to the handicapped or supply an alternative approach to their services. To accomplish this they can redesign their equipment, reassign services to accessible buildings, assign aides to assist the handicapped, make home visits, or deliver services at alternate accessible sites.

Hospitals and other deliverers of services with fewer than 15 persons associated with the operation are exempted from the requirements if providing access to the handicapped would significantly impair their ability to provide services to others. The law provides that if these small facilities find they cannot make a program or activity accessible without a significant alteration of the existing facilities, they may refer the handicapped person to another provider whose services are more accessible.

This law also gives protection to persons handicapped by impaired vision or hearing. Hospitals may not deny these persons benefits or services, give them unequal benefits or services, or provide such services in a way that limits the participation of the handicapped. Furthermore, they must adopt and implement procedures to ensure that persons with such handicaps are able to find out about the services, activities, and facilities available to them.

In addition, hospitals giving notice about benefits or services, or providing written materials about waiver of rights or consent to treatment, are required to ensure that the handicapped are not denied effective notice. Thus the hospital must ensure not only that the information is provided, but that it is received. This part of the law also applies to those with impaired sensory or speaking skills. For example, a hospital that receives federal funds must establish a procedure for effective communication with persons with impaired sensory perception. The institution has the responsibility to provide interpreters who can use sign language, or employ such auxiliary aids as Braille and taped materials for persons with impaired sensory (hearing or vision), manual, or speaking skills.

The regulations to implement the Rehabilitation Act of 1973 are enforced by HHS for health institutions such as hospitals. The regulations spell out the steps the facilities must take to provide accessibility.

Subpart C of the Code of Federal Regulations Sec. 84.52 specifically refers to emergency health care. It states: "A recipient hospital that provides health services or benefits is to establish a procedure for effective communication with persons with impaired hearing to provide emergency health care."

Thus policies and procedures written for emergency departments should include provisions for the treatment of the handicapped. Problems such as accessibility and communication require careful attention.

In 1977 the law was upheld by the courts in *Halderman* v. *Pennhurst State School and Hospital,* 446 F. Supp. 1295 (D.C. Pa., 1977). This suit was brought by former and present retarded residents of the named institution, charging that, because of staff shortages, they were denied access to proper education, training, and rehabilitation. The court agreed that retarded individuals met the law's definition of handicapped persons and should, therefore, not be subject to discrimination in treatment.

The plaintiffs' basic complaints revolved around lack of treatment due to staff shortages. Among their complaints were the following: only one-third of residents requiring physical therapy were receiving it; no long- or short-term goals for residents were set; no communication classes were offered; physical restraints and psychotropic drugs were used for control purposes; seclusion rooms were used for punishment; many residents suffered injuries because of lack of supervision. Administrative personnel were not held monetarily liable as they had made a good faith effort to provide needed service but were unable to do so because of lack of staff.

The facility was ordered to provide access to treatment by removing the residents from its institution to community living arrangements and other community services that could provide minimally adequate habilitation for the residents.

Part V

Administrative Issues

Chapter 10

Administration in General

A hospital can provide adequate medical staff for its emergency department in a variety of ways: hiring salaried physicians, requiring all members of the hospital medical staff to cover the emergency department under some type of rotation plan, or contracting with an independent group of physicians to serve as medical personnel for the emergency room. In many states statutes or regulations require that the emergency department provide at least a specified minimum amount of physician coverage. A failure to provide appropriate staff and facilities for emergency service, where the hospital is under legal obligation to furnish emergency care, could result in hospital liability if such failure caused harm to a patient. Hospital liability could be predicated on corporate negligence for failure to provide necessary services, or it could be based on the application of respondeat superior for the acts of personnel who sought to provide attention but did so in a negligent fashion.

Under respondeat superior, for the hospital to be liable for a physician's malpractice in the emergency room, the hospital must have some control over the work performed; a physician's membership on the hospital's medical staff alone would not be sufficient to lead to the imposition of liability. Thus, where a physician is summoned to the hospital to render care in the emergency room, under a rotation agreement among members of the medical staff, the hospital would ordinarily not be responsible for that doctor's acts. However, some courts may take the position that when the physician has been assigned to the emergency room by the administration, and the appearance of a master-servant relationship is created by the hospital personnel, liability may be imposed on the hospital under respondeat superior for harm suffered by the patient.

A hospital that contracts with a partnership of physicians to provide 24-hour emergency room care, and does not retain the right to direct the specific medical techniques used by physicians, will ordinarily not be liable for negligent treatment rendered by the physicians.

In a Georgia case, *Pogue* v. *Hospital Authority of DeKalb County,* 120 Ga. 230, 170 S.E. 2d 53 (1969), the complaint alleged that a patient in the defendant hospital had died as the result of negligent treatment received from an emergency department physician acting as a servant of the hospital. The court, after examining the contract between the hospital and the physician, determined that the agreement expressly designated the physician as an independent contractor. In affirming a judgment for the hospital, the court held:

> A hospital is not liable for the negligence of a physician employed by it where the negligence relates to a matter of professional judgment on the part of the physician when the hospital does not exercise and has no right to exercise control in the diagnosis or treatment of illness or injury.
> *Pogue* v. *Hospital Authority of DeKalb County,* 170 S.E. 2d at 54.

Contract provisions dealing with the duties of the physicians, delineating which patients the physicians will treat, making clear the standard of medical practice to be provided, and explaining that treatment will be under the surveillance of the hospital's medical staff do not necessarily constitute control by the hospital sufficient to modify the independent contractor relationship set forth in the contract.

Whether the hospital has exercised the requisite control over the emergency department physician is a question of fact that must be determined according to the facts as they are presented in each case.

Recent cases indicate that the courts are inclined to give less weight to the provisions of "insulating" contracts between the hospital and contracting emergency room physicians; the courts are inclined to hold both the hospitals and those physicians liable on the basis of the public's reliance on the hospital and its chosen professional personnel.

The Joint Commission on Accreditation of Hospitals' (JCAH's) Accreditation Manual sets forth procedures and criteria that hospitals should use in granting physicians staff privileges. According to the manual, "[T]he medical staff shall ensure that each [physician] is qualified for membership and shall strive to maintain the optimal level of professional performance of its members . . . ."[1] Accordingly, JCAH requires a reasonably comprehensive delineation of each member's privileges and some evidence of demonstrated competence at the time of admission. Prospective members are obligated to complete an application form containing information required by the hospital's medical staff bylaws. They are also asked to disclose any successful or currently pending challenges against their license to practice medicine, any prior loss of medical society or hospital staff privileges, and any adverse malpractice action.

The medical staff is further requested to act upon the application within the time frame specified in the medical staff bylaws.

Staff privileges, JCAH states, should not be granted to a physician merely because he or she is licensed in a state to practice medicine, is a member of a professional organization, or has staff privileges elsewhere. Specialty board certification is, however, an "excellent benchmark to serve as a basis for privilege delineation."[2]

Physicians and dentists who have contracted to provide emergency room services for a hospital must, as must all applicants, satisfy medical staff requirements and be staff members. Finally, all physicians applying for hospital staff privileges are regarded by the JCAH as implicitly consenting, by virtue of the applications, to the hospital's inspection of all documents related to their qualifications.

Hospital governing boards and medical staff appoint various committees to carry out the business of governing and operating the hospital. The credentials or privileges committee is one of the committees that may collect confidential information in order to fulfill its responsibility to review physicians for appointment or reappointment to the medical staff. Commonly, the medical staff credentials committee will have gathered data about a physician and will make a recommendation to the governing board's committee. Sometimes these reports will contain information about the physician's treatment of particular patients.

These proceedings are subject to several kinds of legal problems. First, if a physician is denied privileges at the hospital she or he may choose to challenge that decision in court and seek to subpoena the committee records. Ordinarily the physician will succeed in obtaining those records for the purpose of the lawsuit. California and Illinois statutes make inhouse hospital committee reports strictly confidential, but provide an exception when a physician's staff privileges are questioned. In connection with the review of a surgeon's deficient performance by the medical staff executive committee, the question arose in *Klinge* v. *Lutheran Medical Center,* 518 S.W. 2d 157 (Mo., 1974), whether the records of the physician's patients could be examined. Over the physician's objection that the physician-patient privilege prevented it, the court found no difficulty in allowing an internal hospital review of those records. It also noted that JCAH standards, state regulations, and Medicare conditions of participation all allowed the use of patients' records in evaluating quality of care.

Second, several states—including New York, Montana, and Georgia—have enacted statutes requiring that reports be made to the medical licensing board about information that appears to show that a physician is medically incompetent, mentally or physically unable to safely engage in the practice of medicine, or is guilty of unprofessional conduct. Failure to report is penalized by suspending or revoking the license of the physician, hospital, insurer, or medical association that does not report as required. Persons who make these reports in good faith are protected from civil and criminal liability. The New York statute specifically declares that this disclosure does not violate the physician-patient privilege.

Third, there has been a considerable amount of litigation over the question of whether the work of medical staff committees, particularly utilization review and other peer review committees, should remain confidential. In order to counter the trend of court decisions that granted patients and other plaintiffs access to these records by subpoena, legislatures have been enacting provisions that protect these committee proceedings from discovery. A related question often arises about the right of patients bringing suits to inspect hospital incident reports. Some hospital attorneys have argued that this file is part of the attorney's "work product" and therefore privileged. In *Hospital Corporation of America* v. *Dixon,* 330 So. 2d 737 (Fla. Dist. Ct. App., 1976), the court held that patients do have the right to see the incident reports unless the hospital can produce sufficient evidence to support nondisclosure. Some statutes now also protect incident reports from discovery.

Fourth, unauthorized disclosure of hospital or medical staff records that might tend to injure a physician's reputation in the community could invite a defamation suit by the affected physician. If the hospital acted out of malice, the doctor might recover for defamation in some states even if the charges were based in fact. Conceivably, public dissemination of the unfavorable information could constitute grounds for a lawsuit claiming invasion of privacy.

In order to avoid some of these problems that can accompany appointment or reappointment procedures, a physician could be required to sign a document authorizing the hospital and medical staff to release any information made in connection with the consideration of the appointment. This release could specify that the members of the medical staff, the hospital governing board, and the hospital administration are allowed to make statements affecting the consideration of the appointment, and that a record of the deliberations can be released to others with a legitimate interest (such as another hospital where the physician is seeking employment).

This release would not bind any patient about whom information was disclosed in connection with the appointment process. Thus, the release does not prevent a patient (as it does the physician) from suing the hospital. Hospital boards and medical staffs should therefore act prudently in handling patients' information during the consideration of physician appointments as well as during peer review and inhouse disciplinary actions.

JOINT COMMISSION ON ACCREDITATION OF HOSPITAL STANDARDS

The Joint Commission on Accreditation of Hospitals has made recommendations in response to the need for more effective emergency services. When required by the complexity of service, the JCAH recommends establishing an emergency department within an existing medical staff, led by a chief who is a member of the medical staff. The chief would be responsible for implementing the policies of the emergency department and for supervising the professional medical services.

Currently JCAH has five standards for emergency services:[3]

Standard I. "A well-defined plan for emergency care, based on community need and on the capability of the hospital, shall exist within every hospital."

Whether the hospital operates no emergency service, a limited one, or a full emergency service, the hospital must have some procedure whereby the emergency patient can be assessed and given "essential life-saving measures and provide[d] emergency procedures that will minimize aggravation of the condition during transportation." The receiving institution must consent to accept the patient before transfer can take place. A reasonable medical record of the immediate medical problem must accompany the patient. Hospitals in a community should identify the readiness of each hospital and staff to receive and treat all emergency patients.

Standard II. "The emergency service, when maintained, shall be well organized, properly directed, and integrated with other departments of the hospital. Staffing shall be related to the scope and nature of the needs anticipated and the services offered."

There must be an organizational plan that identifies the emergency service and its relationship within the hospital and to other community emergency services. There should be someone who acts as a chief of emergency service. Service must be available 24 hours a day. Coverage by medical staff must be adequate to ensure that an emergency patient will be seen within a reasonable length of time and that any necessary laboratory work will be carried out promptly. Specialists in limited practice must be available on an established schedule for consultation and special services in response to the needs of emergency patients. There should be an adequate number of nurses for the amount and type of care to be provided. These nurses should have been specially trained. Physicians, nurses, and all allied health personnel are required to have cardiopulmonary resuscitative training. The hospital should provide emergency care conferences for ambulance and emergency service personnel and medical staff.

Standard III. "Facilities for the emergency service shall be such as to ensure effective care of the patient."

The emergency service area should be near the emergency entrance and should be easily accessible from within the hospital. The receiving area should be unobstructed, and the service area should have adequate space. Enough reception, examination, treatment, and observation rooms should be provided to ensure effective patient care. Procedures should be designed to eliminate the possibility of contamination and cross-infection, due to the many different diseases that pass through this area. It is preferable that there be separate rooms for urgent limited surgery and for the treatment of fractures, and that there be a separate area for severely traumatized patients.

Instruments and supplies such as drugs, plasma substitutes, and so forth must be on hand for immediate use. All resuscitation equipment and supplies must be suitable for adults, children, and infants.

Suction and oxygen equipment and cardiopulmonary resuscitation units must be available and ready for use. Clinical and radiologic laboratory facilities should be available at all times, and patients should be escorted for tests and radiological services whenever necessary.

If possible, emergency personnel should prepare in advance for the arrival of a critical patient. This preparation can be aided by a communications system between the emergency room and persons at the scene of the accident or in the ambulance. In addition, there must be rapid communication between the emergency service and all functionally related areas of the hospital such as the blood storage area, the surgical suite, clinical laboratories, and diagnostic radiology.

Standard IV. "Emergency patient care shall be guided by written policies and shall be supported by appropriate procedure manuals and reference material."

Policies concerning the extent of treatment to be carried out in the emergency room must be periodically reviewed, revised, and approved by the medical staff and the hospital management. Procedures should be developed from the policies. JCAH lists minimum policies and procedures that should be maintained.

Current toxicology reference material is to be readily available, as well as the telephone number of the regional poison control center. Charts detailing the initial treatment of burns, cardiopulmonary resuscitation, and tetanus immunization should be displayed.

Standard V. "A medical record shall be kept for every patient receiving emergency service; it shall become an official hospital record."

The record must contain adequate patient identification; the time and means of arrival and by whom transported; the history of the injury or illness, including first aid administered prior to arrival at the hospital; a description of any findings; diagnosis and treatment; final disposition of the patient (including instructions given); and the condition of the patient on discharge or transfer. The record is to be signed by the physician in attendance. A control register should be kept. The emergency room medical records should be used to evaluate the quality of emergency medical care on a regular basis.

JCAH standards are quasi-legal standards and could establish duties that would then result in liability for negligence if adopted but ignored by a hospital. In *Board of Trustees of Memorial Hospital* v. *Pratt,* 72 Wyo. 120, 262 P. 2d 682 (1953), the chairman of the hospital's credentials committee had recommended to the board of trustees that Dr. Pratt not be reappointed as a member of the hospital's medical staff unless he brought his records up to date to the satisfaction of the records committee. Both JCAH and several state licensing regulations specifically required prompt completion of records after the discharge of patients. The board of trustees, as plaintiff, asked the court for a declaratory judgment and decree to the effect that the rules and regulations adopted by the board of trustees and the medical staff in regard to recordkeeping were reasonable, and that if Dr. Pratt did not comply with these rules he should permanently be enjoined from making use of the facilities. A state statute had made the board responsible for keeping records, and the board had promulgated its recording requirements under delegation of power from this statute. The board of trustees won the case.

Standard II of the JCAH standards addresses the organization and management of emergency services. This is important in terms of providing quality care, as well as in terms of orderly operation. Regardless of whether a brand new emergency department is being organized or an existing service is being enlarged or reorganized, the evaluation and planning should be done by those most involved in the actual giving of emergency care. It is especially important that members of other hospital departments be involved in planning for emergency services. By involving members of other departments, mutually cooperative methods of operation can be worked out prior to implementation of services. For example, the relationship between the emergency physicians and the rest of the hospital medical staff is of crucial importance. When this relationship is tense, because of professional or other reasons, it can lead to problems in patient care and can create an atmosphere of confusion that ultimately could result in negligence and liability.

It is equally important to seek community input wherever practical. Community needs provide the real justification to develop, expand, eliminate, or reduce the delivery of emergency services. Thus, in organizing an emergency department, it is important to have at hand as many relevant facts about community needs as possible.

By studying facts on past utilization, one can determine what kind of program is needed in the future. Any study of utilization should include data on the number of visits, average length of visits, seasonal variations, variations as to time of day and time of week (to show peak and slack hours), and treatment categories. In studying treatment categories, it would be important to see how many cases seen in an emergency department are not of an emergency nature. It would also be important to study the disposition of patients seen for emergency care. A study of actual costs should be made in order to determine charges for service.

Each hospital must study its own situation to determine what kind of emergency department is needed, how to best meet community needs, and how to ensure that quality service is maintained. Clearly, there are many ways to set up an emergency department. Because no two situations are identical, there is no one best plan that would satisfy every situation.

ADMINISTRATION

Different hospitals will have various administrative patterns that dictate the overall management of the institution or facility. The emergency department should be part of this overall administration. The department should be seen and recognized as one of the hospital's more complex, important, and dynamic services. It should be identified as a major service and recognized as important enough to merit administrative time and attention. Regardless of the organizational structure, it is essential that patient-centered care be stressed.

The basic purpose of organization is to ensure that patients are treated promptly and properly by qualified, trained personnel. In a typical emergency service, providing a wide variety of procedures and treatments every working day, it is essential that department personnel be able to function with flexibility, cooperation, and order. To accomplish this, there must be clear lines of authority for administration. The lines of authority should outline areas for clinical practice if these are different from overall management.

Some hospitals have chosen to use an operational committee for management of the emergency services. The operational committee functions under the authority and direction of a larger Professional Advisory Committee for Emergency Care. The advisory committee outlines policies that are to be implemented by the operational committee, whose authority is delegated from the advisory committee.

An operational committee would consist of the Emergency Services Director, the Assistant Administrator of the hospital, the Assistant Director of Nursing with responsibility for emergency services, the Head Nurse of the emergency department, the Chief Physician's Assistant, the Business Manager, and the Social Service Worker assigned to the emergency room. The operational committee would schedule weekly meetings.

The advisory committee, in this management structure, is a much larger body. It consists of all the members of the operational committee as well as the Director of Public Relations, the administrators of the hospital and outpatient clinic, and representatives of all major departments (including anesthesiology, psychiatry, pathology, radiology, gynecology and obstetrics, neurosurgery, orthopedic surgery, and medicine). The main function of this kind of advisory committee is to formulate and recommend policies to guide the administration of the emergency department. In addition, the advisory committee is responsible for utilization review of emergency services and for recommending changes in policies when necessary or desirable. The advisory committee meets monthly.

The administrative management scheme outlined above is but one possible approach; it is not the only way. Each facility should determine, with legal counsel, the best method for administration of not only emergency services but of the entire institution. It is essential, however, that a member of the administrative staff be delegated the responsibility for administrative function designed to address clinical activities. In addition, a member of the medical staff should be designated medical director of the emergency department, with overall responsibility for professional activities within the department.

POLICIES AND PROCEDURES

Emergency department policies and procedures should be formulated and documented in an emergency department manual that is readily available to all staff members of the department. In order to keep the manual current, it should be revised and updated as needed, at least annually.

The policies must clearly reflect the philosophy of the hospital's administrative, nursing, and medical staff. Therefore, preparation of a policy and procedure manual would necessitate the cooperation of members of each of these three disciplines. Because there are many staff members and a large number of services in a typical emergency department, this inevitably results in an equally large number of professional, procedural, and administrative problems. By addressing these issues in a way that is efficient and fair, the emergency department will be able to function well.

Before the policies and procedures can be addressed, the basic questions of philosophy, objectives and goals, function, and attitude must be outlined. Such issues as methods of financing, staff training, and use of health personnel also need to be discussed and resolved.

The policy manual, when drafted and adopted, should function as a resource manual for staff members. It should include information on particular problems that arise in the emergency room, including statements released to the press, interaction with law enforcement officers, interaction with other community agencies, and social service needs.

It is imperative that staff members of the emergency department be familiar with the policies and procedures outlined in the manual. Once policies and procedures are implemented, it is important to obtain feedback from staff on their workability so that appropriate revisions and amendments can be made. The policies must be followed by each and every staff member to ensure effective management of the department.

In formulating policies and procedures, the working committee should involve members of the community whenever possible. This will ensure that the policies address community needs. This is not to say that community members should dominate a drafting committee or dictate to health professionals what services should or should not be offered. But because hospitals are located in many different kinds of communities—some rural, some inner-city, some dominated by a particular cultural or ethnic group—hospitals need community input to ensure that community-identified needs are addressed.

Because emergency room staff deal regularly with such problems as child abuse, injuries that result from criminal activity, and so forth, a number of the policies will have legal implications. Therefore, it is highly advisable to have legal counsel review suggested policies before they are adopted and implemented. It is not important to have a lawyer be a member of the policy-making committee, because many of the procedures and policies do not involve legal questions. Rather, have a lawyer review the entire manual for legal questions. Legal counsel for the hospital would be an appropriate person to perform this crucial task.

STAFFING

The emergency department is one of the greatest points of contact between the hospital and the members of the community it serves. People come to the emergency service in various states of anxiety, fear, and unpreparedness. People in this emotional state may not be able to discuss their situations rationally. It is most important that members of any emergency department be highly skilled and competent. In addition, they should be able to work calmly and

with self-control. All staff members should receive a thorough orientation and training, including training in how to deal effectively with the public. The staff should be able to communicate well with patients and with family and friends who seek relief from fear and anxiety.

Nursing Staff

Emergency department nurses are most often registered nurses, although a large number of licensed practical nurses also staff emergency departments. Emergency department nurses are almost always employees of the institution, as opposed to emergency room physicians who staff in a variety of ways. The role a nurse plays in an emergency setting is very different from the role played by the traditional nurse on a medical-surgical unit. The emergency nurse at various times must institute life-saving measures, perform triage, begin intravenous solutions, and perform a myriad of other highly skillful nursing tasks—many times under great stress.

Nurses hired as staff members of the emergency department should be highly qualified, intelligent, and flexible. Because the emergency nurse has a broad range of responsibilities, she or he should be given corresponding authority. For example, in emergency departments so small that a physician is not on 24-hour duty, nurses must be given authority to begin life-saving measures.

The Emergency Department Nurses Association provides a way for nurses to obtain more knowledge and develop standards for efficient delivery of emergency nursing services. Ongoing education, in the form of workshops and conferences, are provided by this and other associations. Hospitals should encourage emergency staff nurses to keep their knowledge current by giving them time to attend such postgraduate seminars.

For the sake of continuity and most efficient patient care, nurses staffing an emergency service should be permanent members of the department and not rotated from other units in the hospital. As employees of the hospital, nurses are part of service in the emergency department as they are in other departments. Problems involving staffing or any other question should be handled through the lines of authority established in the policy manual.

The number of nurses staffing the emergency department will vary according to patient load. Peak admissions occur from 8:00 A.M. to 8:00 P.M., so staffing should be planned accordingly. Mills, in an article on organization and staffing, called for seven to nine nurses per day for each 100 patients seen, when nursing work shifts were tailored to peak load hours.[4] Each institution has to study its own situation to determine how much staff is needed, but this decision should never be made without consulting those who are best able to advise: the nursing staff of the emergency department.

Physician Staff

As opposed to the nursing staff, which by and large consists of hospital employees hired by the hospital, the medical staff of emergency departments is organized in a variety of ways. In departments with case loads of 20,000 per year or more, Mills has called for a basic physician staff to be on the premises every hour of every day. In high trauma regions, he recommends full staffing as being justified even with a lesser patient load. He then recommends adding one full-time emergency physician for each 7,000 cases seen annually.[5] Adequate staffing of physicians, as with nurses, will vary with each institution. It should be planned, however, in the same way—by looking at the community demand for services and meeting this demand with competent, qualified, skilled physicians.

As with the nursing profession, physicians have formed a national organization, the American College of Emergency Physicians. This organization has developed specialty certification to designate those physicians who have demonstrated by training and examination that they qualify as certified emergency physician specialists.

In the past few years, more than two dozen university programs were offered for formalized residency training in emergency medicine. These graduates are just now entering the field and their impact is beginning to be felt.

Ideally, physicians hired for the emergency department would be those trained in emergency care. However, this is not always possible, especially in small rural hospitals. The governing body of the hospital ultimately must decide what staffing plan is most appropriate, balancing the needs of the community it serves against the availability of physicians.

The Accreditation Manual for Hospitals, on medical staffing for emergency departments, states:

> Service must be available 24 hours a day, and medical staff coverage
> must be adequate to ensure that an applicant for treatment will be
> seen within a reasonable length of time relative to his illness or injury.
> If laboratory procedures are indicated and ordered, due regard must
> be given to promptness in carrying them out. Additional members
> of the medical staff shall be on call for consultation and for unusual
> contingencies. The services of specialists should be made available by
> prearrangement. Acceptable methods of providing medical coverage
> include the use of house staff under adequate medical staff super-
> vision, rotating panels of staff physicians and contracting groups
> whose members are members of the medical staff.[6]

This language is rather broad but does spell out acceptable methods of physician coverage. Each hospital, after careful study, must determine which method is most appropriate. As the service grows or shrinks and as there is some change in the availability of physicians for coverage, the method of coverage will have to be reexamined and adjusted.

One acceptable method is the concept of full-time emergency physicians with no other practice. This method, called the Alexandria Plan, is an efficient and effective way to organize physician coverage. Introduced in the 1960s, it has proved to be effective where used. The drawback with this plan is that often there were too few physicians able and willing to work as full-time emergency physicians. This resulted in the use of part-time, "moonlighting" physicians or residents, often from other institutions. Thus the continuity this method was designed to achieve was often compromised.

Another method of coverage that has seen wide use involves the rotating of staff members, often called the Pontiac Plan. This method has been used on a voluntary and on a compulsory basis. The rationale behind this method is that physicians should be able to give first aid, provide life-saving measures, and make a tentative diagnosis to refer for additional care. However, the drawback of this plan proved to be that there were great disparities in skill as physicians took their turns in rotation.

A newer method is a variation of the Alexandria Plan. Full-time physician coverage is provided by a partnership or corporation of four or five licensed physicians who sign a contract with the hospital. This method can work well if the contract very clearly delineates the responsibilities as well as the authority of the contracting physicians. With this method, coverage is assured. Furthermore, the liability for acts of negligence would be with the contracting physicians only, as independent contractors, because they are not employees of the institution. Thus respondeat superior would not apply. In this situation patients should be notified that they will be billed separately by the physicians for their services, since the physicians are working as independent contractors. If the contracting physicians maintain a private practice in addition to their contract with the hospital, the practice should be kept separate from coverage of the emergency department.

An even newer method is presently evolving, mainly in large metropolitan areas—the multihospital emergency physician group. These groups are large, comprising 50 or 60 physicians. Because emergency medicine is hospital-based, this method offers security to its members. Contracts are established, usually on an annual basis. Thus if one contract is not renewed, the renewal of other contracts compensates. If this method works well for the physicians, it also offers security for the hospital because the emergency physicians do not develop their own private practices. Instead, their work helps build the hospital's emergency department practice.

Still another method used by hospitals involves using residents and interns under the direction and supervision of staff physicians. With this method, the lines of authority and chains of command should be clearly delineated and understood. With residents who do not have a good command of English—especially in hospitals with large numbers of patients who do not speak English as their first language—very close supervision should be provided to eliminate problems resulting from language barriers, especially as related to instructions, referral, and consent.

If the hospital chooses to staff its emergency department with house officers, the governing body of the hospital must remember that their skill varies widely. As employees of the hospital they are not independent contractors, and so the hospital's exposure for liability is increased. Their work must be supervised carefully.

The policy manual should delineate the responsibilities of both house and attending staff when both are used. If medical students are used in addition to residents and interns, the policy manual should state clearly who is responsible for their supervision.

Yeargin et al. v. *Hamilton Memorial Hospital,* 229 Ga. 870, 195 S.E. 2d 8 (1972), demonstrates the court's willingness to uphold the rules and regulations a hospital establishes to provide adequate medical coverage for its emergency department. The facts revealed that Hamilton Memorial Hospital regularly employed four doctors for emergency service. In September 1971, when this suit was filed by Dr. Yeargin, only two doctors were so employed, despite a vigorous recruitment program and search for additional doctors. The case arose from Dr. Yeargin's refusal to accept assignment to the emergency room service as required under the "By-laws, Rules and Regulations" of "The Medical and Dental Staff of Hamilton Memorial Hospital." Dr. Yeargin sued the hospital for damages and an injunction to prevent it from denying him access to and the use of the hospital for his patients. He contended that compelling him to work in the emergency room against his will was arbitrary, unreasonable, and a violation of the Fifth, Thirteenth, and Fourteenth Amendments to the U.S. Constitution. The trial court denied a temporary injunction. This decision was appealed.

The court reviewed the rules and regulations and found they were neither arbitrary, unreasonable, discriminatory, nor unconstitutional. The court pointed out that Dr. Yeargin had been assigned four days of "back-up" duty in September, the month in which he brought suit. The purpose of such duty was to assist the regularly employed emergency doctors in the event of their illness or overload of seriously ill emergency patients, or to assist in providing specialty treatment, admission of patients to the hospital, and follow-up treatment. There was evidence that emergency room duty such as Dr. Yeargin's required on the average of one and one-half hours of service per week. The evidence also showed that in December 1971, the hospital had regularly employed three doctors for emergency patients and had expected to employ a fourth physician by March 1972. Dr. Yeargin testified that he had performed emergency room service over the past 20 years, but that he was now physically unable to do so. He stated that he treated between 1,800 and 2,000 of his own patients each month and had worked for 22 months, seven days a week, without a vacation. However, he had had a complete physical examination on October 15, 1970, and was certified as physically fit; his airplane pilot's license had been approved. He stated that his general health had not changed since then, except that he was older and more tired. At the time of the suit, Dr. Yeargin was 54 years of age; the medical staff rules excused doctors from emergency service at age 60.

The court stated that contrary to Dr. Yeargin's assertion, he was not compelled to perform emergency room service against his will. He was only required to perform reasonable emergency room service in order to use the facilities of the Hamilton Memorial Hospital. These facilities were available to him, but only upon his acceptance of the corresponding burden of reasonable service for emergency duty.

The court then affirmed the lower court's judgment by holding that Dr. Yeargin's rights had been scrupulously observed during the hospital's administrative proceedings and the proceedings of the trial court, and that a hospital authority may restrict a staff member's privileges by reasonable and nondiscriminatory rules and regulations.

Two cases with somewhat similar causes of action produced different results based on the facts in each case. Both cases involved the use of unlicensed emergency room physicians. In the earlier case, *Rush* v. *Akron General Hospital,* 171 N.E. 2d 378 (Intermediate App. Ct., Ohio, 1957), the unlicensed physician was hired by the hospital as an intern. The court pointed out that the intern was a medical college graduate and licensed to practice medicine in the state of Wisconsin but was not licensed to so practice in the state of Ohio. At the time of the events giving rise to this case, the intern was on a "twenty-four hour tour of duty" to serve patients coming to or brought to the hospital's emergency room. In the action against the hospital for negligence, the plaintiff claimed that the hospital was negligent, in that its servant—the doctor—closed a wound without probing it, thereby leaving in the patient's back two small pieces of glass.

The court pointed out that negligence cannot be found simply because the intern was not licensed. The court stated that the great weight of authority supports the view that a failure to procure a license does not in itself give rise to any right of recovery by the plaintiff. To maintain such an action, the court said, the plaintiff must show that the result complained of was due to negligence or unskillful treatment. The court rendered judgment for the hospital, stating that the plaintiff's claims were not supported by the necessary proof, especially since the senior staff member of the hospital—an eminent surgeon—had examined the plaintiff two days after the emergency treatment and found nothing to indicate glass in the wound.

In the later case, *State Board of Medical Examiners* v. *Warren Hospital,* 102 N.J. Super. 407, 246 A. 2d 78 (1968), there was no issue of negligence. The State Board of Medical Examiners, as plaintiff, brought suit for a penalty alleging that Warren Hospital, as defendant, violated a New Jersey statute by employing an unlicensed physician in the emergency room. The physician was licensed in Pennsylvania but not in New Jersey where he was working. The defendant hospital claimed that the statute only applied to the practice of medicine by individuals, and the state legislature never intended that the legislation regulate hospitals. The court rejected the defendant's contention, stating that the section prohibiting the practice of medicine without a license did apply to hospitals since that was the intent of the legislature. The court held that the defendant was in violation of the New Jersey statute and was therefore subject to the mandatory penalty provided. It rendered judgment for the plaintiff in the sum of $200.00, the statutory penalty.

Joining a growing nationwide trend, the U.S. Court of Appeals for the Eighth Circuit in *Balhuizen* v. *North Kansas City Memorial Hospital,* 8th Circuit, August 8, 1978, validated a private hospital's right to maintain a "closed staff" for selected medical departments. Although this ruling did not involve an emergency service, an analogy can be made. The ruling involved a staff physician who maintained a subspecialty in pulmonary diseases but was denied continued full access to the hospital's Inhalation Therapy and Pulmonary Department laboratory. The ruling followed the facility's decision to designate another physician as the individual exclusively charged with operating the laboratory. The excluded physician argued that this arrangement, which as a practical matter prevented other physicians from administering pulmonary tests or interpreting their results, violated his rights of due process and equal protection under the Fourteenth Amendment. Noting that he "had not been denied any privileges enjoyed generally" by other hospital physicians and that all staff members were required to abide by this policy, the court concluded that the "closed staff" arrangement infringed upon no federally protected rights.

Elsewhere, in *Lewin* v. *St. Joseph Hospital of Orange,* 82 Cal. App. 3d 368, 146 Cal. Rptr. 892 (1978), a California appeals court similarly refused to strike down a private hospital's decision to retain its renal hemodialysis facility on a "closed staff" basis. The arrangement grants one group of physicians the right to operate this service to the exclusion of all others. One excluded physician unsuccessfully claimed that the arrangement was illegal since it interfered with his practice of medicine and required that any of his patients who wished to undergo treatment in this hospital employ a physician other than himself. Turning this claim aside, the court ruled that it could not be said that the hospital's policy was "substantively irrational . . . or procedurally unfair." Courts should not unduly interfere with a hospital governing board's policy-making decisions. And here, the court reasoned, the board reasonably had determined that a "closed staff" operation facilitated administration of the unit, simplified the scheduling of patient treatment, ensured adequate physician supervision, facilitated supervision and training of nurses and other personnel, and was less costly than alternative treatment procedures. Moreover, it ensured immediate availability of a nephrologist during the 14 hours a day the unit was in operation. Furthermore, there was—at most—minimal interference with the complaining physician's right to practice his profession, as he maintained hemodialysis privileges in numerous other local hospitals.

Thus, in organizing physician staff coverage, it is important to recognize that courts are willing to uphold the rules and regulations of hospitals so long as those rules and regulations are not unreasonably discriminatory. The closed staff concept should be upheld by the courts if used in the staffing of an emergency service, since it has been upheld when used for similar units of service within a hospital.

Additionally, in organizing physician staff coverage, in hiring physicians as hospital employees, or contracting with one or more physicians as independent contractors, the governing body of the hospital must be certain that the contractual arrangements are explicit in the mutual responsibilities of the parties. In *Rucker* v. *High Point Memorial Hospital,* 20 N.C. App. 650, 202 S.E. 2d 610, aff'd, 206 S.E. 2d 196 (1974), the trial court had directed a verdict for the defendant hospital on the basis that the plaintiff had failed to show that the defendant physician was the agent, servant, or employee of the defendant hospital; on the contrary, all the evidence showed that defendant Dr. Stovall was an independent contractor. The appellate court disagreed. It reviewed the contract between hospital and physician that had been introduced into evidence by the plaintiff. Under the contractual terms, the physician had been guaranteed an annual salary as a member of a four-person team to work in the emergency room. All fees in excess of the guaranteed salary would be divided among the physicians. In addition, the physicians had agreed to phase out their private practices within one year, and they had agreed to not accept other work in their off-duty hours (which would have amounted to going into private practice in competition with members of the active medical staff). The court stated that this contract clearly created an employment relationship and not that of an independent contractor. The court then held that the trial court had erred in directing a verdict against plaintiff in favor of defendant, and for this and other reasons ordered a new trial.

The responsibilities of emergency physicians should be detailed in policies and procedures, and these should be followed. At a minimum, physician responsibilities should include the following: to be available at all times while assigned to the emergency room; to give proper and prompt care at all times; to treat patients in order of urgency; to assume full responsibility for patients until other arrangements or adequate referral has been made; to be certain that any referral will not harm the patient's chances of recovery or will not cause an existing condition to further deteriorate; and to complete a detailed, concise, accurate, and legible record on each patient seen, stating what specific actions were taken and why.

Other Personnel

Many other types of health personnel are currently used in emergency departments of general hospitals to allow for effective management and operation of the service. Social workers can be highly effective in helping with referrals for home care, counseling, and public assistance. They can also be utilized for on-the-spot counseling for patients, family, and friends.

Physicians' assistants are currently used in many emergency departments. Legally, the physician's assistant is an extension of the physician and must work under the direct supervision of a doctor. Their use in the emergency room is legally the same as in any other service.

The physician's assistant is a new development in health care. At present, training programs vary a great deal—from courses of a few weeks or months to degree-granting courses. Hospitals using physician's assistants must be just as careful delineating their responsibilities, duties, and authority as they are with all their employees.

As the reader can see, the efficient administration of the emergency departments of general hospitals requires compliance with a myriad set of statutes, regulations, and judicial decisions. The establishment and maintenance of internal policies to ensure such compliance should relieve emergency room staff members of concern about legal complications and allow them to concentrate on what they do best: care for their patients.

NOTES

1. Joint Commission on Accreditation of Hospitals, *Accreditation Manual for Hospitals,* February 1978 ed. (Chicago: JCAH, 1978), p. 73.

2. Ibid., pp. 74-75.

3. Ibid., pp. 15-19.

4. James D. Mills, "The Emergency Department: Organization and Staffing," in *Principles and Practices of Emergency Medicine,* Vol. II, George Schwartz et al. (eds.), (Philadelphia, London, Toronto: W. B. Saunders Co., 1978), pp. 1440-1443.

5. Ibid.

6. Joint Commission on Accreditation of Hospital Standards in *Emergency Medical Services Workbook,* (Germantown, Md.: Aspen Systems Corporation, February 1978), pp. 5-4 to 5-15.

Glossary of Legal Terms

Abandonment: Legally, termination of the physician-patient relationship by the physician without the patient's consent or without the patient being given sufficient time or opportunity to obtain the service of another physician.

Abortion: The termination of pregnancy or the inducement of a termination of pregnancy.

Administrative agency: An arm of government that administers or carries out legislation; for example, the Workmen's Compensation Commission.

Admissibility (of evidence): Worthiness of evidence that meets the legal rules of evidence and therefore will be allowed to be presented to the jury.

Affidavit: A voluntary sworn statement of facts, or a voluntary declaration in writing of facts, that a person swears to be true before an official authorized to administer an oath.

Agency: A relationship in which one person acts for or represents another; for example, the employer and employee relationship. (Employers can be held liable for the acts of their employees acting as their agents.)

Allegation: A statement that a person expects to be able to prove.

Appellant: The party who appeals the decision of a lower court to a higher jurisdiction.

Appellee: The party against whom an appeal to a higher court is taken.

Arteriogram: An x-ray picture of an artery after the injection of a contrast medium into it.

Assault: An intentional act designed to make the victim fearful and produce reasonable apprehension of harm.

Assignment: A transfer of rights or property.

Attestation: An indication by a witness that the documents of procedures required by law have been signed.

Battery: The touching of one person by another without permission.

Best evidence rule: The legal doctrine requiring that primary evidence of a fact (such as an original document) be introduced, or at least explained, before a copy can be introduced or testimony given concerning the fact.

Bona fide: In good faith: openly, honestly, or innocently; without knowledge or intent of fraud.

Borrowed servant: An employee temporarily under the control of another. The traditional example is a nurse employed by a hospital who is "borrowed" by a surgeon in the operating room. The temporary employer of the borrowed servant will be held responsible for the act of the borrowed servant under the doctrine of respondeat superior.

Civil law: The laws of a state or nation regulating ordinary private matters (distinguished from criminal, military, or political matters).

Common law: The legal traditions of England and the United States where part of the law is developed through court decisions.

Concurring opinion: *See Opinion of the court.*

Confidential information: *See Privileged communication.*

Consent: A voluntary act by which one person agrees to allow someone else to do something. For medical liability purposes, consents should be in writing with an explanation of the procedures to be performed.

Contusion: A bruise.

Coroner's jury: A special jury called by a coroner to determine whether the evidence concerning the cause of a death indicates that the death was brought about by criminal means.

Counterclaim: A defendant's claim against a plaintiff.

Crime: An act against society in violation of the law. Crimes are prosecuted by, and in the name of, the state.

Criminal law: The division of the law dealing with crime and with punishment by the state. A person can be punished under the criminal law by the state and sued under the civil law by the victim for the same act. For example, an assault case can appear in civil and criminal court.

Curettage: The process of removing diseased tissue from body cavities such as the uterus with a scoop-shaped surgical instrument.

Decedent: A deceased person.

Defamation: The injury of a person's reputation or character by willful and malicious statements made to a third person. Defamation includes both libel (written) and slander (oral).

Defendant: In a criminal case, the person accused of committing a crime. In a civil suit, the party against whom suit is brought demanding compensation to the other party.

Deposition: A witness' sworn statement, made out of court, which may be admitted into evidence if it is impossible for the witness to attend in person.

Directed verdict: The verdict returned by a jury when the judge directs the jury to return a verdict in favor of one party because the evidence or law is so clearly in favor of one party that it is pointless for the trial to proceed further.

Discovery: Pretrial activities of attorneys to determine what evidence the opposing side will present if the case comes to trial. Discovery prevents attorneys from being surprised during a trial and facilitates out-of-court settlement.

Dissenting opinion: *See Opinion of the court.*

Emancipation: Termination of parental control over a minor and parental legal duty to support the minor.

Emergency: An emergency is any condition that—in the opinion of the patient, his family, or whoever assumes the responsibility of bringing the patient to the hospital— requires immediate medical attention. This condition continues until a determination has been made by a health care professional that the patient's life or well-being is not threatened. *True emergency:* A true emergency is any condition *clinically* determined to require *immediate* medical care. Such conditions range from those requiring extensive immediate care and admission to the hospital to those that are diagnostic problems and may or may not require admission after work-up and observation.

Emergency care system: The term emergency care system denotes a community or regional network of services that provides for detection and reporting of medical emergencies, initial care at the scene, transportation and care en route to a medical facility, and care of the patient until he or she is discharged, referred, or admitted for definitive medical care.

Emergent: Requires immediate medical attention. Delay is harmful to the patient. Disorder is acute and potentially threatens life or function.

Employee: One who works for another in return for pay.

Employer: A person or firm that selects employees, pays their salaries or wages, retains the power of dismissal, and can control the employees' conduct during working hours.

Expert witness: One who has special training, experience, skill, and knowledge in a relevant area and who is allowed to offer an opinion, based on that training, experience, etc., as testimony in court.

Federal question: A legal question involving the U.S. Constitution or a statute enacted by Congress.

Felony: A crime of a serious nature usually punishable by imprisonment for a period of longer than one year.

Fistula: An abnormal passage leading from an abscessed cavity or a hollow organ such as a vagina to another organ or to the skin's surface.

Gastrointestinal: Gastroenteric; relating to both the stomach and intestine.

Good samaritan law: A legal doctrine designed to protect those who stop to render aid in an emergency.

Grand jury: A jury called to determine whether there is sufficient evidence that a crime has been committed to justify bringing a case to trial. It is not the jury before which the case is tried to determine guilt or innocence.

Grand larceny: The theft of property valued at more than a specified amount (usually 50 dollars), thus constituting a felony instead of a misdemeanor.

Harm or injury: Any wrong or damage done to another, either to the person, or to the person's rights or property.

Hearsay rule: A rule of evidence that restricts the admissibility of evidence that is not the personal knowledge of the witness. Thus, an out-of-court statement cannot be used to prove the truth of the statement except under certain limited circumstances.

Hematoma: A swelling filled with extra vasated blood. *Subdural hematoma:* hematoma beneath the dura matter (a membrane forming the outer envelope of the brain).

Holographic will: A will handwritten by the testator. It is valid only in some states.

Hospital: An organizational entity composed of a governing board, a staff (medical and nonmedical), and an administrative structure. The term hospital applies to that entire organizational entity.

Hospital emergency department: A hospital's facilities and services provided primarily for the management of outpatients who come to the hospital for treatment of conditions determined clinically or considered by the patient or his representative to require immediate medical care in the hospital environment. The term is synonymous with emergency room, accident room, and casualty room.

In loco parentis: The legal doctrine providing that, under certain circumstances, the courts may assign a person to stand in the place of a minor's parents and possess their legal rights, duties, and responsibilities for that minor.

Indemnity: Legal exemption from penalties attaching to illegal actions granted to public officers and other persons.

Independent contractor: One who agrees to undertake work without being under the direct control or direction of an employer.

Indictment: A formal written accusation of crime brought by a prosecuting attorney against one charged with criminal conduct.

Injunction: A court order requiring one to do or not to do a certain act.

Interrogatories: A list of questions to be answered sent from one party in a lawsuit to the other party.

Intracranial: Within the skull.

Judge: An officer who is authorized to hear and determine cases in a court of law. He or she also guides court proceedings to ensure impartiality and enforce the rules of evidence. The *trial judge* determines the applicable law and states it to the jury. The *appellate judge* hears appeals and renders decisions concerning the application of the law to the case.

Jurisprudence: The philosophy or science of law upon which a particular legal system is built.

Jury: A certain number of persons selected and sworn to hear the evidence and determine the facts in the case.

Larceny: The taking of another person's property without consent and with the intent of depriving the owner of its use and ownership.

Leading Case: A case often referred to by the courts and by counsel as having finally settled and determined a point of law.

Liability: An obligation one has incurred or might incur through any act or failure to act.

Liability insurance: A contract to have someone else pay for any liability or loss thereby in return for the payment of premiums.

Libel: A false or malicious writing that is intended to defame or dishonor another person and is published so that someone besides the one defamed will observe it.

License: A permit from the state allowing certain acts to be performed, usually for a specific period of time.

Litigation: A trial in court to determine legal issues, rights, and duties between the parties to the litigation.

Malpractice: Professional misconduct, negligent discharge of professional duties, or failure to meet the standard of care of a professional that resulted in harm to another.

Mastectomy: Amputation of the breast.

Misdemeanor: An unlawful act of a less serious nature than a felony, usually punishable by fine or by imprisonment for a term of less than one year.

Negligence: Carelessness; failure to act as an ordinary prudent person, or action contrary to the conduct of a reasonable person; action or nonaction by a professional person contrary to that of a reasonable, prudent, professional person.

Next of kin: Those persons who by the law of descent would be adjudged the closest blood relatives of the decedent.

Non compos mentis: "Not of sound mind;" suffering from some form of mental defect.

Nonurgent: Not requiring the resources of an emergency service. Disorder is minor or nonacute.

Notary public: A public official who administers oaths and certifies the validity of documents.

Nuncupative will: An oral statement intended as a last will made in anticipation of death. It is valid only in some states.

Opinion of the court: In an appellate court a statement of its decision. One judge writes the opinion for the majority of the court. Judges who agree with the result (but for different reasons) may write *concurring opinions* explaining their reasons. Judges who disagree with the majority may write *dissenting opinions.*

Ordinance: A law passed by a municipal legislative body.

Perjury: The willful act of giving false testimony under oath.

Petit larceny: The theft of property usually valued at below 50 dollars and classed as a misdemeanor.

Phenylketonuria: Congenital deficiency causing brain damage.

Plaintiff: The party to a civil suit who brings the suit seeking damages or other legal relief.

Podiatrist: Specialist in the diagnosis and treatment of the human foot.

Police power: The power of the state to protect the health, safety, morals, and general welfare of its citizens.

Precedent: A court, in making a decision, will try to follow principles used in previous decisions where the facts raise similar issues.

Privileged communication: A statement made to an attorney, physician, or certain other people in a position of trust. Because of the confidential nature of such information, the law protects it from being revealed, even in court. Thus, the communications between certain persons, such as physician and patient, cannot be divulged without the consent of the patient. In some situations the law provides an exemption from liability for disclosing information where there is a higher duty to speak, such as statutory reporting requirements. Valid only in some states.

Probate: The judicial proceeding that determines the existence and validity of a will.

Probate court: A court with jurisdiction over wills and certain other matters depending upon the law of the particular state.

Proprietary hospital: Private hospital, operated for profit.

Proximate: In immediate relation with something else. In negligence cases, the careless act must be the proximate cause of injury.

Real evidence: Evidence furnished by tangible things, such as weapons, bullets, and equipment.

Rebuttal: The giving of evidence to contradict the effect of evidence introduced by the opposing party.

Regulations: Rules of a governmental agency that have the force of law and are written to implement a law.

Regulatory agency: An arm of the government that enforces legislation regulating an act or activity in a particular area; for example, the federal Food and Drug Administration.

Release: A statement signed by one person relinquishing a right or claim against another person or organization, usually for a valuable consideration.

Res gestae: All of the surrounding events that become part of an incident. If statements are made as part of the incident they are admissible in court as res gestae, as an exception to the hearsay rule.

Res ipsa loquitur: "The thing speaks for itself." A doctrine of law applicable to cases where the defendant had exclusive control of the thing that caused the harm and where the harm ordinarily could not have occurred without negligent conduct, and the plaintiff could not have voluntarily contributed to his or her own injury.

Respondeat superior: "Let the master answer." The legal doctrine that holds the employer responsible for the legal consequences of the acts of the servant, or employee, while acting within the scope of employment.

Saline solution: A salty solution normal to the body.

Slander: An oral statement made with intent to dishonor or defame another person when made in the presence of a third person.

Standard of care: Those acts performed or omitted that an ordinary prudent person or professional would have performed or omitted. It is a measure against which a defendant's conduct is compared.

Stare decisis: "Let the decision stand." The legal principle indicating courts should apply previous decisions to subsequent cases involving similar facts and legal issues.

State statute; statutory law: A declaration of the legislative branch of government having the force of law.

Strict liability: Liability without regard to fault; absolute liability for an injury.

Subpoena: A court order requiring one to appear in court to give testimony.

Subpoena duces tecum: A subpoena that commands a person to come to court and to produce whatever documents are named in the order.

Subrogation: The substitution of one person for another in reference to a lawful claim or right.

Suit: A court proceeding in which one person seeks damages or other legal remedies from another. The term is not usually used in criminal cases.

Summary judgment: A judgment rendered by a judge for a plaintiff upon the failure of a defendant to controvert the plaintiff's motion sufficiently to show the existence of a genuine issue of fact.

Summons: A court order that directs a sheriff to notify the defendant in a civil suit that a suit has been filed and when and where the defendant is to appear.

Testimony: The oral statement of a witness given under oath at a trial.

Tort: A civil wrong. Torts may be intentional or unintentional.

Tortfeasor: One who commits a tort.

Triage: Prompt, brief clinical evaluation of all incoming patients to determine the nature of the problem, the level of urgency, the identification of the kind of service needed, and assignment for emergency attention.

Trial court: The court in which evidence is presented to a judge or jury for decision.

Urgent: Requires medical attention within a few hours. In danger if not attended. Disorder is acute but not necessarily severe.

Verdict: The formal declaration of a jury's findings of fact, signed by the jury foreman and presented to the court.

Vicarious liability: One is held responsible for another's liability. For example, under the doctrine of respondeat superior, employers are held liable for the negligent behavior of their employees.

Waiver: The intentional giving up of a right, such as allowing another person to testify to information that would ordinarily be protected as a privileged communication.

Will: A legal declaration of the intentions a person wishes to have carried out after death concerning property, children, and estate.

Written authorization: A consent given in writing specifically empowering someone to do something.

Table of Cases

Index

I

Imprisonment, false. *See* False
  imprisonment
Incident reports, 214
Incompetence (mental). *See* Mental
  incompetence
Incompetence (physician), 213-14
Independent contractors
  administration and, 211-12, 223,
    227
  law of agency and, 26
  respondeat superior and, 27, 28,
    32-33, 35-36
  statute of limitations and, 38
Informed consent. *See* Consent
  (informed)
Instruments, 9, 216
Intentional wrongs, 6
Interns, 73, 85, 110, 111, 144
  autopsy and, 130
  emergency staffing and, 224
  respondeat superior and, 29, 30
  staffing/negligence and, 225-26
Interpreters. *See* Translators
Intoxicated patients. *See* Patients,
  drunken
Intrauterine device (IUD). *See*
  Contraceptives

J

Joint Commission of Accreditation
  of Hospitals
  admissions and, 75
  autopsy and, 130
  emergency care standards of, 7-10,
    215-18
  physician's staff privileges and,
    212-13
  recordkeeping and, 171
  transfer standards and, 106

L

Laboratory facilities, 9

Law. *See also* Reporting laws
  adult protection, 164-65
  autopsy consent, 132-34
  common, 17
    defined, 3-4
    emergency admissions and, 75,
      76
  consent and, 87-88
  criminal, defined, 5-7
  regulations and, 4, 5
  state, discrimination and, 194
  statutory
    admissions and, 82-83
    defined, 4
    discharge and, 139
  tort
    defined, 5-7
    law of agency and, 26

Law of agency, 26, 28, 33
Law enforcement officers. *See* Police
Leprosy, 156
Levels of care, 10
Liability
  blood transfusions and, 11-13
  consent and, 89, 93, 98, 99, 103
  contracts and, 223
  discharge and, 138, 141, 151
  emergency departments exposure
    to, 52-53
  intentional wrongs and, 6
  malpractice and, 15-23
  negligence and, 13-15, 17, 18, 19,
    20, 21, 22, 23, 23-27, 29-30, 32,
    33, 34, 35, 36-38
  overview of, 10-11
  possession of body and, 127
  psychiatric patients and, 151
  res ipsa loquitur and, 23-25
  respondeat superior and, 13, 25,
    26, 27-34
  staffing and, 211
  statute of limitations and, 38-40
  strict, 11-13
  transfer delay and, 105
  vicarious, 25-38

M

Malpractice, 52, 99, 148, 211, 212
212
  admissions policies and, 85
  anesthetics and, 24
  breach of contract and, 37
  criminal law and, 5-6
  "discovery" rule and, 39, 40
  independent contractors and, 32, 33
  liability and, 15-23
  res ipsa loquitur and, 25
  statute of limitations and, 38-40
  as tort action, 13
Massachusetts Civil Rights Act, 195
Medicaid
  federal/hospital regulations and, 170-71, 205
  handicapped patients and, 169
Medical examiner
  cases of, 120-21
  DOA cases and, 119-20
  reporting laws and, 160
Medical records, 14
  abortion/reporting laws and, 159
  births out of wedlock and, 159-60
  consent and, 56-57, 93-94
  discharge and, 138
  DOA cases and, 120
  drugs and, 168
  emergency commitment and, 150
  hospital, reporting laws and, 170-72
  JCAH standards and, 9, 10, 216-17
  rape cases and, 65
  reportable diseases and, 156
Medicare
  federal grants/hospital regulations and, 170-71, 194, 205
  handicapped patients and, 169
  patient care and, 213
Meniscocytosis (sickle cell anemia), 158-59
Mental illness

consent and, 104
discharge and, 148-49, 150, 151
emergency admissions and, 148-49
false imprisonment and, 7
transfer and, 105
Mental incompetence, consent and, 103-104
Midwives, 159
Minors, consent and, 89, 93, 99-101
Moral neglect, child abuse reporting and, 163
Multi-level care. *See* Levels of care

N

Neglected children, consent and, 101. *See also* Child abuse
Negligence
  admissions and, 78, 79, 80
  blood transfusions and, 11-13
  causation and, 17-21
  consent and, 91
  contracts and, 223
  corporate, 13-14, 15, 26-27
  damages and, 21-23
  discharge and, 136, 138, 141, 143, 145
  liability and, 11, 13-15
  malpractice and, 15, 17, 18, 19, 20, 21, 22, 23
  possession of dead body and, 127, 128
  recordkeeping and, 172
  res ipsa loquitur and, 23-25
  staffing and, 225-26
  statute of limitations and, 38-40
  transfer and, 108
  vicarious liability and, 25-27, 29-30, 32, 33, 34, 35, 36-38
Newborns. *See* Birth
Nurses, 14, 144, 150, 152
  administration and, 215, 221
  admissions examples and, 72-73, 74, 77-78, 196-97
  consent and, 92-93
  drugs and, 168

149-51
gunshot wounds and, 160-61
as independent contractor, 28,
  32-33, 35-36, 38, 211-12, 223,
  227
new drugs and, 167
patients of private, admission and,
  50-51, 81, 145
records and, 217
refusal of emergency room service
  and, 224-25
reporting laws and, 156-159
respondeat superior and, 28, 32-36
selection of, 14-15
staff, admission of patients of,
  51-52, 69, 85
staff privileges and, 212-14, 225
triage and, 45-46
Physician's assistants, 228
Poison control center, 9, 216
Poisonings, reporting of, 161
Police, 144
child abuse cases and, 140, 163
discharge and, 136
sexual assault cases and, 65
tests/consent and, 59, 60
wounds/reporting laws and,
  160-61
Policies and procedures
administrative, 219-20, 224
admissions and, 85-86
consent, 94
death and, 130
debt collection, 204
discharge and, 138
drugs and, 166
efficiency and, 52
elective, discouraging, 53
emergency commitment, 53
handicapped patients and, 206
hospital, defined, 4-5
reporting laws and, 156, 161
transfer/abandonment and, 113
written, JCAH standards and, 9,
  216
Pontiac Plan (emergency

physicians), 223
Post-mortem examination, 120, 130.
  See also Autopsy
Precedent, 3-4
Procedures. *See* Policies and
  procedures
Professional Advisory Committee,
  218-19
Proximate cause, 18, 19, 20, 21, 22,
  34, 149. *See also* Causation
Psychiatric patient. *See* Mental
  illness
Psychiatric work
elective, 53
the handicapped and, 205
Public Health Service. *See* United
  States Public Health
  Service

Q

Quarantine, 157

R

Rape, 63-65, 161
Records. *See* Medical records
Regulations
federal
  civil rights and, 194-97
  Hill-Burton Act of 1946 and,
    198-204
  hospital records and, 170-71
  overview of, 193
  Rehabilitation Act of 1973 and,
    204-207
governmental agency, 4-5
Rehabilitation Act of 1973, 169,
  204-207
Reliance, theory of, 50-51, 197
Reporting Laws. *See also* Laws
abused children and, 155, 161-63
births/deaths and, 159-60
criminal acts and, 160-61
diseases and, 156-59
drug laws and, 155, 166-69

About the Authors

MARGUERITE R. MANCINI is both a registered nurse and a practicing attorney, one of only a few individuals in this country to successfully combine these two fields. She is a member of the bar in the state of Connecticut. She has held many nursing positions and has taught nursing as well. Among her responsibilities was the supervision of nursing students in the emergency room setting. She has written a regular column for *The American Journal of Nursing* on legal issues in nursing. In addition, she has conducted seminars around the country on nursing and the law and has served as a legal consultant to *Nursing 81* and to state agencies in Connecticut.

After earning an undergraduate degree in education, ALICE T. GALE received her J.D. from the University of Connecticut School of Law. She has taught on various levels in several states and is currently a general practitioner of law in Danbury, Connecticut. She has combined teaching and law by instructing adult education classes in legal issues.